THE NEMECHEK PROTOCOL FOR AUTISM AND DEVELOPMENTAL DISORDERS

THE HOW-TO GUIDE TO RESTORING NEUROLOGICAL FUNCTION (2ND EDITION)

PATRICK M. NEMECHEK, D.O.

JEAN R. NEMECHEK, J.D.

AUTONOMIC RECOVERY, LLC

CONTENTS

PART III

VAGUS NERVE STIMULATION

PART IV
THE UPS AND DOWNS OF RECOVERY

PART V
THE SCIENCE BEHIND THE NEMECHEK PROTOCOL®

PART VI
THINKING ABOUT THE FUTURE

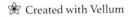 Created with Vellum

ACKNOWLEDGMENTS

My path of professional education and personal enlightenment has traveled through the seemingly diverse medical fields of HIV disease, the autonomic nervous system, and chronic inflammation only to discover the body's enormous capacity to recover from past insults and prevent future maladies.

Through a combination of perseverance and the guidance of others who have had a substantial impact on advancing medicine (Einstein, Feingold, Tracey), I pressed forward to find new approaches that genuinely improve health rather than simply masking disease.

I can think of the many times I might have given up and simply become another typical clinic doctor if it were not for the support of so many patients willing to try something new. I have asked many patients to try a new approach only to have it fail but yet, undeterred, they return asking me to try again.

Occasionally our combined efforts would be successful, and we would then work on improving their condition even further. From learning to control the ravages of wasting syndrome in HIV disease to reversing chronic brain injuries, and finally to help children develop neurologically, I would not have been nearly as successful without the faith and support of my patients and their parents.

Beyond working with patients, constantly operating outside the traditional medical community is at times emotionally exhausting and professionally isolating. As they say, the last mile of any journey is the hardest, and it has been my wife Jean's love and faith in our shared purpose that has helped me press forward.

She is my most trusted counselor and my unwavering source of support and love. Without her, I would have never been able to finish the last mile of my journey.

Thank you, everyone, for your support.

Patrick Nemechek

MEDICAL DISCLAIMER

The information and the images contained within this publication are provided as an informational resource only and are not to be used or relied on for any diagnostic or medical or treatment purposes.

This information is not intended to be patient education and does not create any patient-physician relationship.

Please consult with a licensed healthcare practitioner to determine if any of these therapeutic approaches are appropriate for you or your child.

INTRODUCTION

A NEW ERA OF OPTIMISM FOR BRAIN RECOVERY

Fifteen years ago, when I began my research on the autonomic nervous system (ANS), my research was turning up some strange findings regarding neurological recovery after a common concussion. I was seeing many adults who had experienced mild to moderate concussions several years prior but who were still experiencing neurological symptoms from the accident along with testing abnormalities of their ANS.

I found this puzzling because there are studies from the 1960's that indicated as long as someone did not bleed within their brain from their injury, they should fully recover within about three months. In other words, if your concussion was so severe you were knocked unconscious for several minutes, you were expected to fully recover within a few months.

I was perplexed that these people not recovering.

At the time that I began investigating brain injuries, the prevailing scientific view was that after we are born our body was no longer capable of producing new stem cells nor new neurons. This meant that there was very little capacity for the brain to recover from injury.

In other words, if a person did not spontaneously recover from a brain injury there was little hope of any further recovery.

This confused me because thirty to forty years earlier it was assumed the brain was fully capable of recovery. Now the brain was viewed as the least capable organ of recovery. Nevertheless, I pushed on with my efforts to try and help these patients somehow recover from their autonomic dysfunction.

The First Breakthrough in Recovery

For the first few years, I had minimal success in helping patients improve both symptomatically and objectively on their tests looking at autonomic functioning (known as spectral analysis). I was trying a wide variety of neuroplasticity techniques with little results.

Then a succession of scientific papers from 2008-2012 began to paint a picture that in fact, humans do produce stem cells not only after birth but throughout our entire lifespan. The only problem was that chronic inflammatory stress prevented these stem cells from working.

This was a critically important finding for me because stem cells were also being viewed as vital to the body's natural repair and rejuvenation mechanisms. I decided upon a rather simplistic strategy. I thought that if I could lower inflammation enough in my patients, their naturally produced stem cells might be activated enough to allow their brain to naturally repair their old injuries.

I set about trying a variety of supplements and lifestyle changes that I felt would lower inflammation within the brain. Within a few months, patients began to report significant improvements in their symptoms. These same patients were also finally demonstrating neurological recovery on their autonomic tests.

Over the following years, I did countless little studies comparing supplements and lifestyle changes with respect to their potency in improving symptoms and test results. The result is the present version of The Nemechek Protocol®. Yet some of the unbelievable recoveries I was seeing still seemed impossible, even with healthy functioning stem cells.

The Second Breakthrough in Recovery

Although we had clear evidence that the human body actively produced stem cells, there was little to no evidence that neurons were being replaced with healthy new neurons. It was hard for me to believe that stem cells alone were responsible for the unbelievable recoveries that were occurring.

My skepticism finally resolved in 2019 with the discovery that an important region of the adult brain called the hippocampus was replacing 90% of all its neurons with new healthy neurons every three weeks. The hippocampus is an important region of the brain in regard to cognition, memory, and emotionality.

Additional proof of the nervous systems regenerative capacity came from studies indicating that the five hundred million neurons found within the intestinal tract were also replacing 90% of themselves every two weeks.

So, it seems like the 1960's viewpoint of the brain's ability to fully recover from most injuries was correct. The only difference between the 1960's and now is that most people now are experiencing chronic inflammation and their stem cells, repair, and rejuvenation mechanisms are unable to function quickly.

Medical science is finally re-discovering that the human brain is designed by nature to fully and rapidly repair itself from all but the most severe brain injuries. With this knowledge, I started suggesting similar strategies to patients with children afflicted with a variety of childhood conditions such as autism, developmental delay, intestinal distress, failure to thrive, anxiety, sensory processing disorders, low motor tone and even cerebral palsy.

Over the following years, several incremental changes have refined the original anti-inflammatory protocol and is now known as The

Nemechek Protocol®. The protocol is ground-breaking and original that a patent (U.S. #10, 335,396) was issued in July 2019 for *Methods of Reversing Autonomic Nervous System Damage.*

My anti-inflammatory protocol was then modified for use in children after I discovered it was also effective in helping children to recover from autism, developmental delay, as well as a wide variety of symptoms resulting from unrepaired common brain injuries.

The unexpected success and wide application of my discovery has brought us to this point, The Nemechek Protocol® as it applies to children. May this book explain the root of many problems and a way to achieve healing across the globe forever more.

PART I

HOW TO START THE NEMECHEK PROTOCOL®

1

NEWFOUND OPTIMISM IN THE HOPE FOR RECOVERY

Many parents have experienced the crushing news that their child has autism and that there is little hope of recovery. Parents are counseled not to expect too much for their child's future. They are not encouraged to be hopeful for a neurotypical child and that such hope for a neurotypical child is beyond realistic expectations. Years of neuroplastic drilling might help improve some behaviors but often with very minimal standards to consider something a success.

The reason for such pessimism is that most physicians and therapists are still operating from the old paradigm that the brain cannot recover. What is worse yet, many do not realize that their efforts directed at helping their child are bridled by the fact they have been trained that there is little hope for recovery.

If someone believes there is little chance to change a situation, their efforts at changing the situation often become half-hearted or non-existent. Therefore, if physicians never whole-heartedly try to help patients recover from a chronic brain injury, they likely will never have their patients recover.

The cycle of low expectations, minimal effort, and minimal success reinforces the physicians' belief that they were correct in not trying help the brain to recover.

This belief structure is referred to as a self-fulling prophecy, a scenario with overriding implications in our efforts to help children with autism and developmental issues.

The modern fact is that in the absence of chronic inflammation that prevents proper brain development and healing from injuries, the vast majority of children with autism and developmental issues should spontaneously recover from any neurological injury or insult they experience. Their neuronal repair and rejuvenation mechanisms should continue them on the path of normal neurological recovery.

I think this optimism also applies to children who have a genetically-based diagnosis for their neurological challenges. I admit that a reduction of inflammation will not reverse the anatomical abnormalities some children display from their genetic disorder, but I have witnessed profound neurological improvements in these same children whose hope for any form of improvement or recovery was deemed impossible.

Recent scientific advances are teaching us that the brain is capable of fully repairing severe injuries, producing stem cells, and is continually replacing neurons throughout life.

These discoveries are painting a picture that instead of being incapable of recovery, the human brain is perhaps the *most capable* organ of recovery after insults or injuries. And in my experience, chronic inflammatory stress is the single most likely culprit to inhibit recovery.

Inflammation is a normal process in which white blood cells in the body become activated to fight infections and repair tissue. Inflammation is turned on, resolves the problem at hand, and then is naturally turned off. If it is short-lived and regulated properly, inflammation promotes health throughout our lives.

4

But, if inflammation is running continually in an unregulated fashion, inflammation will cause damage throughout the body by a direct toxic effect on the tissues as well as by inhibiting some of the body's other natural repair mechanisms.

Sources of unnatural inflammation can be found in many aspects of our environment. Polluted air, changes in our food supply, chronic psychological stress, and alterations in our intestinal bacteria all contribute to increasing levels of inflammatory stress within our body.

Knowing that inflammation is the key to many of our health problems, my first priority for my patients is to first lower inflammation. By recreating balance in fatty acid nutrients we give our brain and nervous system, by balancing bacterial overgrowth in our intestinal tracts, by avoiding inflammatory oils in modern foods, and by bioelectric stimulation of the autonomic nervous system when necessary, the stage is set for improvement and recovery for a wide range of childhood and adult ailments.

2

THE NEMECHEK PROTOCOL® OVERVIEW

The Basic Science (The Short Version)

There is growing scientific evidence that an imbalance of intestinal bacteria alongside excessive inflammation in the brain may be responsible for the features associated with autism, developmental delay, and mood disorders.

Furthermore, brain injuries from even minor head traumas in children cannot be completely repaired and these result in other common symptoms such as constipation, hyperactivity, anxiety, aggression, poor focus, fatigue, and insomnia.

The Nemechek Protocol® as it relates to children begins with a simple two-pronged approach that involves restoring proper balance of intestinal bacteria along with a restoring a normal ratio of omega-3 and omega-6 fatty acids.

Eliminating inflammation from these sources re-activates natural brain repair and pruning mechanisms, often leading to substantial recovery from developmental delay and previously unrepaired brain injuries.

The reduction of inflammation is primarily achieved by rebalancing intestinal bacteria and balancing the intakes of omega-3 and omega-6 fatty acids.

Continue reading through this chapter to understand the key points of the protocol. Specific dosing instructions for each component of the protocol I use with my patients will be provided.

More detailed explanations of these steps will be presented in greater detail in later chapters for those who want a deeper understanding of the science behind the protocol.

First Step – Reduce Bacterial Overgrowth within the Small Intestine

The most important barrier to overcome when considering brain function health is the presence of excessive colonic bacteria within the small intestine.

Known as small intestine bacterial overgrowth (SIBO), bacterial overgrowth triggers the release of a large wave of inflammatory chemicals that prevent the brain from developing normally. Overcoming SIBO is the single most important step in helping a child to recover.

To emphasize the difference between the bacteria within the small intestine compared to the bacteria within the colon (also referred to as the lower or large intestine), there's an analogy I use: think of the bacteria from the colon as "fish" and the bacteria from the small intestine as "birds."

With SIBO, the fish are living up in the small intestine with the birds. Everyone knows that fish and birds are two very different animals and that they are not meant to live side-by-side together.

The following diagram shows the ideal balance of fish and birds with each living within their respective environments. The small intestine has very few bacteria compared to the colon.

For every individual "bird" bacterium in the upper small intestine, there are one hundred million "fish" bacteria living in the lowest portion of the colon; an enormous 1:100,000,000 difference in bacterial concentrations.

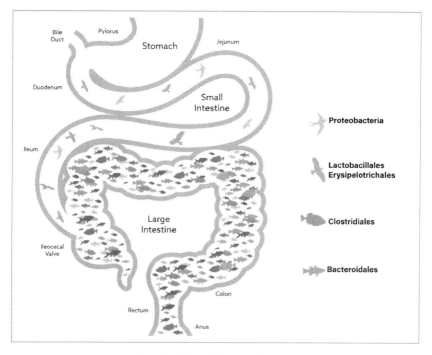

Normally Balanced Intestinal Bacteria

Bacterial overgrowth occurs when a single species of "fish" bacteria migrates up from the colon and begin replicating within the small intestine. The overgrowth from the invading bacteria results in one thousand to one hundred thousand times the normal bacteria within the small intestine.

Medical science has been aware of bacterial overgrowth within the small intestine for approximately sixty years. This is not a new discovery and many decades of scientific research have been devoted to methods to help rebalance intestinal bacteria.

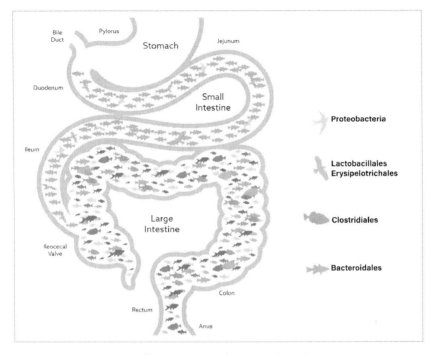

Small Intestine Bacterial Overgrowth (SIBO)

The excessive numbers of bacteria in the small intestine overwhelm its ability to properly contain its contents and small fragments of bacteria and food molecules leak into the surrounding tissue. The failure to contain the contents is scientifically known as bacterial translocation but is more generally referred to as "leaky gut."

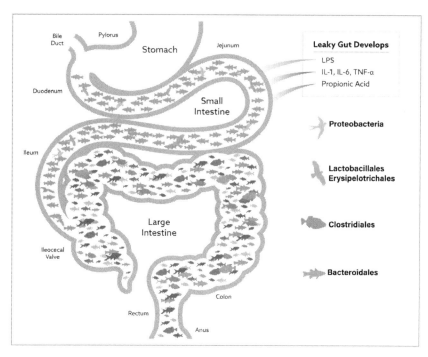

SIBO Leads to Leaky Gut (Bacterial Translocation)

The tissue surrounding the small intestine contains approximately eighty percent of all white blood cells within the body. The leakage of bacterial cell wall fragments (LPS) and food molecules are viewed as foreign to the white blood cells and result in a very large inflammatory reaction releasing inflammatory chemicals into the blood stream.

Known as cytokines, these inflammatory chemicals flow throughout the body and into the brain where they prevent the brain from normally developing by interfering with normal neuronal pruning and repair mechanisms.

Of the thousand or more different species of bacteria ("fish") that normally live within the colon, overgrowth most often only occurs when one unique species fish bacteria starts living with the birds.

Occasionally, the overgrowing fish bacteria within the small intestine are also capable of producing large amounts of a chemical called propionic acid.

When large quantities of propionic acid leak into the bloodstream, it can have a sedating effect on children, which makes them behave as if they are drugged or heavily medicated. It is the sedating effect of propionic acid that is responsible for kids losing eye contact, not responding readily, and generally behaving with very little awareness of their surroundings.

The Nemechek Protocol® uses an over-the-counter prebiotic fiber called inulin to balance the bacteria in younger children, and a non-absorbable antibiotic called rifaximin to balance the bacteria in older children and adults. Reversal of bacterial overgrowth by either method leads to a rapid decline in systemic inflammation and brings the excessive production of propionic acid to a halt.

Within a few weeks of reversing bacterial overgrowth, the small intestine will naturally heal itself leading to a rapid decline in the release of inflammatory cytokines and propionic acid. Rifaximin and inulin are not to be used in combination.

Once bacterial overgrowth is reversed and propionic acid levels decline, these children are released from the toxic, stuporous prison they have been trapped in. Within a few days they often become more aware, have improved eye contact, and respond more readily to their name or simple commands. I refer to this early response as "the awakening period." The awakening period is a direct effect of the drop in production of propionic acid.

Older children and adults with autism, as well as children with developmental delay but without an autism diagnosis, tend to have little to no awakening period. I believe this is because the bacteria overgrowing in their intestines are probably not capable of producing propionic acid or the propionic acid has less of a negative effect on their nervous system.

If a patient does not experience an awakening, it does not mean the protocol is not working. It simply means they have bacterial over-growth with bacteria that do not produce propionic acid.

Second Step – Rebalance the Intake of Omega-3 and Omega-6 Fatty Acids

Excessive levels of inflammatory chemicals known as cytokines prevent the normal repair and pruning mechanisms of the brain from operating correctly. Balancing the intestinal bacteria has a substantial effect on lowering inflammation but improving the balance of omega-3 and omega-6 fatty acids is also required to allow the brain to recover.

Omega-6 fatty acids are natural chemicals found in plants and are required to activate healthy levels of inflammation to repair tissue or fight infection in the body. Omega-3 fatty acids are natural chemicals found in plants and animal flesh and act as a counterbalance to help turn off inflammation after it is no longer necessary.

Unfortunately, our modern food supply contains an excessive amount of inflammation-promoting omega-6 fatty acids and deficient amounts of inflammation extinguishing omega-3 fatty acids.

An excessive amount of the omega-6 fatty acid chemical called linoleic acid is present in the food supply in the form of vegetable oils, shortening, and the meat from animals who are fed grains such as corn or soybeans.

Fortunately, another tool in the fight against inflammatory omega-6 fatty acids is oleic acid, a fatty acid found in high concentrations in extra virgin olive oil. Oleic acid is able to neutralize the toxicity of excessive linoleic acid. Consuming extra virgin olive oil (EVOO) every day will protect the body from excessive linoleic acid and reduce its negative inflammatory effect throughout the body and brain.

Increasing the intake of omega-3 fatty acids is easily achieved by daily supplementation with fish oil. Although nuts and flax also contain omega-3 fatty acids, two omega-3 fatty acids referred to as EPA and DHA are found in high concentrations fish oil and cannot readily be supplemented in any other manner.

Because of the high frequency of fraudulent fish oil and low-quality olive oil in the marketplace, careful attention must be made to use the correct brands of fish oil and extra virgin olive oil.

3
___

STARTING THE NEMECHEK PROTOCOL

How Early Can The Nemechek Protocol® Be Started?

I recommend that people consult their pediatrician if their child is less than 12 months of age, if there are any other complicated medical issues for a child of any age, or if the child requires prescription medications on a regular basis prior to starting The Nemechek Protocol® or any other new treatment in a child.

I suggest that my patients begin supplementing with fish oil, olive oil, and inulin at the earliest sign of any developmental problems in a child. Starting the protocol in healthy-appearing children can greatly improve their chances of remaining healthy and not developing any developmental issues, cumulative brain injury, or autistic traits.

Day-to-Day on The Nemechek Protocol®

There is no particular order or timing in the day when a parent should administer the inulin, fish oil, or olive oil. They can be taken together or separately, with or without food and in the morning or the evening. While some parents prefer to start just the oils for a few weeks and then add the inulin later, I generally recommend my patients start everything at the same time.

If my patient is older and I am starting with rifaximin instead of inulin, the rifaximin must be taken in divided doses approximately ten-to-twelve hours apart.

I recommend starting with pure organic inulin powder called Nemechek Blue Organic Inulin (NemechekBlue.com) or inulin powder produced by NOW Foods. For fish oil, I recommend a brand of fish oil called Ultimate Omega (liquid or capsule form) produced by Nordic Naturals or DHA-500 also produced by NOW Foods.

Due to the unpredictable quality of extra virgin olive oil found in the market, I recommend using Nemechek Gold (NemechekGold.com) or another California Olive Oil Council (COOC) certified extra virgin olive oil (COOC.com).

I recommend these brands because these are the specific ones I have used with my patients in my office with success over the years. Because of the high level of poor-quality or fraudulent supplements and olive oil in the marketplace, deviating from these options may cause the protocol to fail and prevent the child from recovery.

I also recommend eliminating all additional vitamins, supplements, and remedies unless specifically prescribed by a physician for a diagnosed nutrient deficiency (e.g., iron or Vitamin D deficiency).

First Step - Reduce Bacterial Overgrowth

Ingredient #1 – Inulin or Rifaximin

The prebiotic fiber inulin and the prescription medication rifaximin (Xifaxan®) are my two options to balance the intestinal bacteria. Starting the protocol with inulin is my preferred approach in younger children while I prefer starting with rifaximin in older children because inulin is less effective in older children.

Choosing Between Inulin versus Rifaximin

- If under 8 years of age, I use inulin to balance intestine bacteria
- If between 8-14 years old, I may start with either inulin or rifaximin
- If 15 years of age or older, I recommend starting with rifaximin

Inulin Dosage

- Give a 1/8 teaspoon of powdered inulin
- Can be mixed in food or drink
- Dosage does not change with age

Rifaximin (Xifaxan®) Dosage

- 550 mg twice daily for 10 days
- Medication can be crushed and mixed with food or drink if necessary
- This is a prescription medication and must be obtained through a physician

See chapters 4-8 for more information on using inulin or rifaximin to reduce small intestinal bacterial overgrowth.

Second Step - Rebalance Fatty Acids

Ingredient #2 – Daily Extra Virgin Olive Oil

I only use California olive oil that is COOC-certified and have my patients consume the olive oil daily in its raw and uncooked form either straight like medicine or mixed in food or drink. The minimum required amount of olive oil is listed below.

Under 2 years of age: cook food daily in EVOO

Between 2 to 4 years old: ¼-½ of a teaspoon (1.25-2.5 ml)

Between 4 to 8 years old: 1 teaspoon (5 ml)

Between 9 to 12 years old: 2 teaspoons (10 ml)

Between 13 to 17 years old: 1 tablespoon (15 ml)

18 years or older: 2 tablespoons (30 ml)

Olive Oil Dosages

A listing of COOC-certified olive oils can be found in the appendix and at COOC.com. I have found that it is easier for families to buy the olive oil online direct from a small, regional olive farmer if COOC-certified olive oil is not available in the local market. Nemechek Gold is a phenol rich COOC-certified extra virgin olive oil blended with your child's health in mind. Read more about it at NemechekGold.com.

Ingredient #3 – Daily Liquid Fish Oil

When starting I often recommend the liquid form of fish oil produced by Nordic Naturals called Ultimate Omega (NNUO).

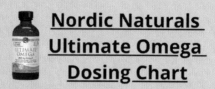

Nordic Naturals Ultimate Omega Dosing Chart

Under 1: Consult with pediatrician about giving daily fish oil

1 to 2 years of age: 1/8 teaspoon (0.6 ml)

3 to 5 years old: 1/4 teaspoon (1.25 ml)

6 to 10 years old: 1/2 teaspoon (2.5 ml)

11 to 14 years old: 1 teaspoon (5 ml)

15 to 17 years old: 2 teaspoons (10 ml)

18 years or older: 1 tablespoon (15 ml)

Fish Oil Dosages

What to Expect with The Nemechek Protocol®

Within the first few weeks of starting, many children may demonstrate much greater eye contact and an improved sense of awareness and connectedness. This is because the sedating effects of propionic acid have been reduced or eliminated due to a rebalancing of the intestinal bacteria. See chapter sixteen for a more in-depth explanation of bacterial overgrowth and propionic acid.

Eliminating the sedative effect will also give a child's parent a sense of potentially how neurologically imbalanced their child actually is. Some behaviors may seem worse because the propionic acid was suppressing their ability to act out these behaviors as a drug might. Such behaviors might be stimming, anxiety, aggression, hyperactivity or sleeplessness. Parents are now seeing their child for the first time without the child being sedated.

In other words, a child's behavior may initially worsen but that does not mean the protocol is not working, it means we have discovered a key to the potential recovery and the starting point we begin working from.

Within the following weeks to months, parents often begin noticing improvements in many aspects of any neurological impairment or delay their child has been experiencing. Although the pace may seem slower than one might have hoped, the recovery marches forward very consistently.

Patience on the parents' part is essential because there is no method to get the child to "improve faster" and efforts to do so often lead to progress stopping completely.

If progress does stop or a parent feels their child is not reacting correctly to the protocol, they will need to refer to the later chapters of the book. This chapter is the short version of The Nemechek Protocol® where later chapters go into more detail and are full of information to answer the inevitable questions that will arise as the child's nervous repairs and prunes itself and starts them on a path of true recovery.

PART II

THE FIRST THREE MONTHS

4

EVALUATING PROGRESS

S uccess in neurological improvement and recovery on The Nemechek Protocol® is highly dependent on maintaining a healthy balance of intestinal bacteria. Without this balance, little to no neurological recovery can occur. Lack of recovery is very rarely due to inadequate doses of fish oil or olive oil, so I tell my patients not to adjust the recommended olive or fish oil doses.

In this section I will explain how I determine if progress is occurring, how I make changes if it is not, and how I decide whether or not additional treatment with vagus nerve stimulation is warranted.

The first question I ask when assessing if the protocol is successful with my patient is whether the use of inulin has been effective in rebalancing the intestinal bacteria. If not, inulin needs to be switched to rifaximin. If the child has already been using rifaximin then they will need to be switched from it being used only occasionally ("as needed") to one of the more aggressive cyclic or continuous rifaximin dosing regimens.

The second question I ask is whether neurological recovery is occurring across all neurological areas that seem to be injured, dysfunctional, or delayed. If the child is experiencing only partial improvement (significant improvements in many areas but little to no improvement in a few others), five minutes of daily vagus nerve stimulation is added to further broaden the neurological recovery. A thorough discussion of the science and use of vagus nerve stimulation can be found in chapters 10 and 11.

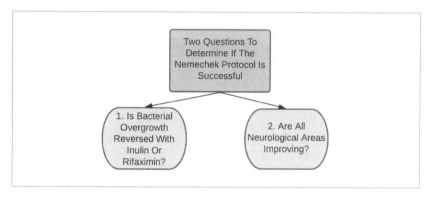

Determining if The Nemechek Protocol is Successful

As simple as this sounds, answering these two questions can sometimes be complicated because many events can occur after starting the protocol that can impede progress and mask recovery but do not indicate improper dosing. Examples might be starting the protocol, but six weeks later the child develops an infection that takes two rounds of antibiotics, and then another four weeks to recover from the effects of the illness and antibiotic treatment for it.

Another example might be that during the first few months of the protocol the family moves and the child experiences many stressors including changing from to different schools with different routines and new teachers and therapists. Both examples are unavoidable situations that can impact recovery, especially early on.

If there are intervening events, the parents and I must account for these and factor them into our decision-making process before deciding if a particular step in the protocol is working or not working.

The Initial Response Patterns to The Nemechek Protocol®

The Nemechek Protocol® may initially bring about two patterns of treatment response within the first three months:

1. Significant improvement in the pace of recovery.
2. Little to no improvement in the pace of recovery.

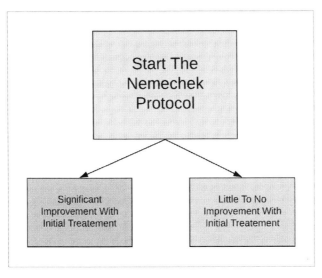

Initial Response Patterns

Making an objective determination about the child's progress is essential in getting the most out of The Nemechek Protocol®.

All aspects of the child's development need to be considered. I take stock of their awareness, emotionality, intestinal function, hyperactivity, social interactions, and motor skills. Sometimes it is helpful for a parent to consult with their child's teachers and therapists about their observations now as compared to when they first started to help determine which response category the child falls into.

Teachers and therapists can be great assistance because their curriculum or programs are often modular in nature with chapters, and skill levels. As professionals who interact with the child frequently, they are in a unique position to observe if the child's pace of learning or developmental improvement has increased or plateaued.

One important thing I tell parents is to not merely focus on their child's ability to speak when determining their progress. It is often the parent's major goal but receptive and expressive communication are possibly the most complex neurological processes we can observe and as such, often take the longest amount of time to observably recover.

Once parents have categorized how well their child has responded to either inulin or rifaximin within the first few months, the remainder of this chapter will help them understand what I do next to maximize their recovery depending on the category they fall into.

The following sections in this chapter are organized based upon my patients' response to treatment. They will either be consistently improving or showing minimal to no response to inulin or rifaximin.

Significant Improvement Scenarios

If inulin or rifaximin is effective in balancing intestinal bacteria and the fish oil and olive oil are dosed properly, parents should observe improvements in multiple areas of development over the first three to six months. The types of improvements include cognition, communication, meaningful play, emotional control, socialization, motor function, and intestinal function and are common in the majority of children I have worked with.

If a significant pace of recovery has begun and the inulin seems to be well-tolerated, there is no need to adjust the dose of inulin, fish oil, or olive oil. The doses of fish oil and olive oil will <u>only</u> need to be adjusted about every one-to-two years as the child ages. The exception is inulin, its dose does not increase over time even with substantial changes in the size or age of the child.

However, in some cases, I have seen improvements that are not uniform across all areas with one or two areas of concern that do not show signs of improvement. Sometimes they may show an initial response that is not maintained with the results proving to be only temporary. Each of these outcomes is shown below.

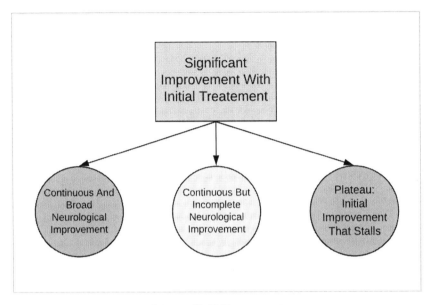

Patterns of Initial Improvement

Little to No Improvement Scenarios

Occasionally it is difficult to see the initial gains in children being treated with inulin because of overlapping anxiety, hyperactivity, and aggression revealed during the awakening. These issues can arise when inulin has effectively stripped away the excessive propionic acid which reveals the true extent of the child's underlying neurological imbalance. In some children the increase in anxiety, aggression, and hyperactivity is so extreme that their inulin must be discontinued.

I refer to this situation as "inulin intolerance." If the increase in these behaviors is tolerable, the inulin can be continued, and the negative behaviors will resolve as the nervous system continues to recover.

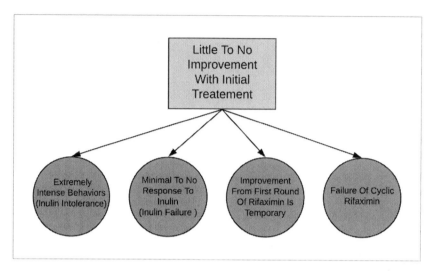

Patterns of Little to No Improvement

If the inulin is well tolerated but there is no significant improvement in the rate of neurological recovery after several months, I consider the inulin to be ineffective and refer to this as "inulin failure."

I have also found that sometimes the child's lack of progress on inulin is due to poor quality or possibly fraudulent inulin. I have had patients who showed no response to the protocol after one year of inulin but suddenly experience an awakening within a few to several days of switching to inulin sold directly from the manufacturer when previously using a non-approved brand or one purchased on a third party website. The same has been true with rifaximin. The authenticity of the product is a variable I must always consider.

And finally, if there is no progress within several months after taking rifaximin, the child is most likely experiencing "rapid rifaximin relapse," and will require either cyclic or continuous rifaximin to maintain a consistent pace of recovery.

5

MANAGING SUCCESSFUL RECOVERY

The most common response to The Nemechek Protocol® is the continuous, broad level state of recovery that can continue on for years. Inulin easily maintains intestinal bacterial balance and protects against relapse despite exposure to antibiotics, intestinal illnesses, anesthesia, slow intestinal motility, and other causes of intestinal bacterial relapse.

For these reasons inulin is my preferred initial method of balancing the intestinal bacteria. The fact that inulin is also inexpensive and readily available worldwide are obvious positive factors as well. Unfortunately, some children may experience inulin failure, a plateauing of their progress when the inulin seemingly fails to work any longer.

Once a child develops inulin failure they will require further treatment with rifaximin to balance their intestinal bacteria. By age fifteen, I will preferentially start children on rifaximin because the chances of lasting response to inulin are very low in my experience.

If rifaximin is not readily available, I recommend starting a child of any age on inulin along with fish oil and olive oil because the combination might still be enough to result in a positive shift in recovery even in older children. Once rifaximin is available, then the inulin can be stopped if it is not effective.

When initially treating with rifaximin parents need to be patient because they may not notice any improvements for four to eight weeks. Because rifaximin is classified as an antibiotic, many parents seem to expect a more rapid recovery, but after either inulin or rifaximin recovery in these children occurs in a slow, continuous fashion. Unlike other antibiotics the parents are familiar with, rifaximin rebalances the intestinal bacteria which allows the nervous system to begin recovering, a process that will continue after the course of rifaximin is completed.

Children initially treated with rifaximin tend to be older, often will have less of a recognizable "awakening," have more developmental delay, a greater degree of maturity delay, and more cumulative brain injuries. For all these reasons older children appear to recover "more slowly" than younger children. The actual truth is the pace of recovery is the same, but the older children just have a greater neurological deficit to recover from.

If the child has been treated with rifaximin, there is a chance that additional treatment with antibiotics, intestinal illnesses, general anesthesia, or slow intestinal motility from underlying autonomic dysfunction may trigger a relapse in intestinal bacterial overgrowth (SIBO) which will halt their recovery.

With a relapse in intestinal bacteria, parents may see a return of some of the symptoms that had been improving after rifaximin or simply an overall plateauing in the pace of their neurological recovery. If there are no other reasonable circumstances to account for the change in behavior, I believe the child will need to be re-treated with rifaximin if the relapse symptoms persist for more than fourteen days.

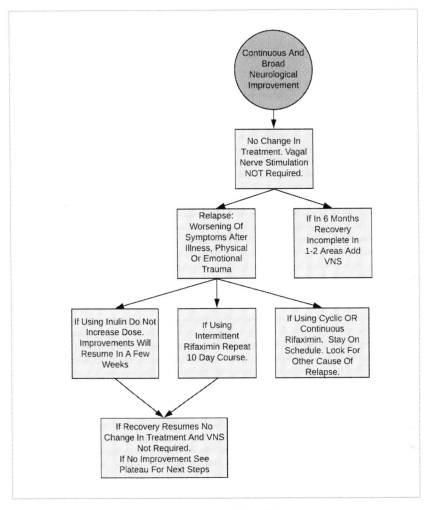

Managing Continuous and Broad Recovery

Waiting approximately fourteen days before repeating rifaximin is necessary because the worsening of symptoms might instead be from a mild intestinal disturbance (virus, medicine, tainted food) or an emotional, physical or inflammatory brain trauma and these would predictably show signs of recovery before the two-week waiting period is complete.

Chronic, low-grade sinus or dental infections are very common events that can cause a temporary and prolonged worsening of symptoms that might be misconstrued as a relapse but in fact, is not. A mild runny nose, cough or flair of allergies can cause enough neurological stress to worsen anxiety, hyperactivity, aggression, and stimming. A simple ten-day course of nasal corticosteroid spray (e.g., OTC fluticasone) can improve the symptoms and lead to a positive trajectory of improvement once again.

Once excessive inflammation is substantially reduced, immune function improves and will begin more effectively clearly areas of low grade infection from the body, especially around the teeth and gums. Increasing dental pain from the improved immune function is also frequent cause of deteriorating behavior, especially if it occurs a month or two after improving balance of intestinal bacteria with rifaximin.

Emotional traumas such as moving into a new home, starting a new school or a change in therapist, increased home stress (pandemic, divorce or separation), and bullying are just a few examples of situations that can cause a temporary halt in recovery. Recovery may not be noticed again until the stress-causing scenario has been dealt with or a new routine is established.

Parents need to monitor all aspects of their child's neurological development to be certain that they are continuing to recover. Sometimes, after four-to-six months parents will realize that their child's recovery was not as complete as is should be or that progress has slowed greatly or even seemed to halt altogether. As stated previously, teachers and therapists can be of great assistance in detecting if the child's progress has hit a plateau.

As shown in the graph below, if a slow, continuous and broad level of neurological recovery is present, no change in treatment is required.

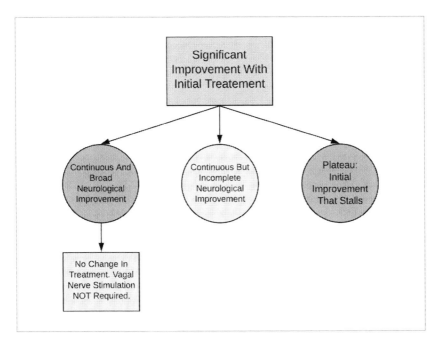

Patterns of Improvement

Sometimes the child will continue to recover but after a few to several months it become apparent that their recovery is incomplete. If incomplete recovery occurs, additional changes to the protocol are then required.

6

RECOVERY PLATEAU

A nother response pattern parents might observe is that the child is experiencing significant improvement, but after several months the pace of recovery dramatically slows and may even stop altogether. Hitting this plateau and it is generally easier to notice than one might think. Parents, therapists, and teachers will often all share the same observation that the child's rate of progress has come to a near standstill.

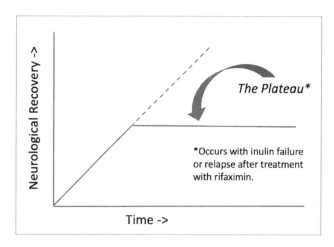

The Recovery Plateau

The first thing I do if I think the patient has plateaued is to look for any new factors that might disrupt intestinal balance or cause new brain trauma. This could be a new supplement or probiotic that has been introduced, a significant new trauma (physical, emotional, or inflammatory), or a new chronic infection such as low-grade sinusitis or a dental infection.

Factors That Interrupt Recovery When Using Inulin

- Physical Brain Injury (concussion, subconcussive event)
- Emotional Trauma (bullying, abrupt routine change, loss of a loved one)
- Inflammatory Trauma (acute infection, surgery, vaccination)
- Recent Infections or Antibiotic Use
- Addition of New Supplement, Remedy
- Addition of Probiotic
- Dental Infection or Pain

Emotional traumas are more common than most parents might believe. I frequently encounter children whose progress is temporarily interrupted because of an emotional event that an adult thinks is minor but is in fact quite significant to the child. I have seen the distress associated with a change in a familiar therapist or teacher, a change in school, bullying or ongoing conflict with peers, a sibling moves out of the home for college, jet lag after a long, difficult flight, or a parent starts traveling for work to be enough trauma to plateau a child's progress for a period of time.

When a plateau occurs, I have my patients stop the use of any supplements, herbal remedies, chelation agents, homeopathic products, or probiotics if they have recently been added. We also treat any potential infections that might exist. Recovery should begin again within a couple of weeks after eliminating the offending event or after the physical or emotional trauma.

I am in complete disagreement with the many "health experts" who recommend probiotics for children and adults in order to improve their gut health. While the concept of simply adding in some "good bacteria" is alluring, the formal medical science regarding gut health does not strongly support the use of probiotics. I personally have cared for patients who have been severely injured by probiotics. In one case, a neurotypical teenager became wheelchair-bound and lost the ability to speak after being prescribed probiotics.

A common source of interference with recovery is a chronic sinus infection that can present subtly with nothing more than a chronic runny nose or a slight cough. Once or twice daily treatment with the OTC nasal corticosteroid fluticasone is a safe and simple treatment remedy for chronic sinus infections and will not disrupt intestinal bacterial balance like common antibiotics might.

As long as the patient is using approved brands of inulin, fish oil, and olive oil, switching brands or making subtle changes in dosage will likely not fix the problem and will often only lead to confusion about the true source of the relapse. The shifts in behavior often noted from these changes were inevitably going to happen whether or not the changes had been made.

Too often I have spoken to parents who began increasing and decreasing dosages after some minor changes in their child's behavior. Quickly changing dosing like this only servers to make the protocol more complex. The parents are confusing common fluctuations in behavior that would eventually correct themselves if nothing were done with a true response to the dose changes.

"The single most important factor resulting in no improvement or a plateau in the rate of improvement is a loss of balance of the intestinal bacteria, not the dose of fish oil or olive oil."

If all efforts to find any ongoing source of interference have failed, it is very likely the bacteria overgrowth of the small intestine has returned despite continued use of inulin and once I have concluded the patient has "inulin failure" I stop the inulin and treat the patient with rifaximin.

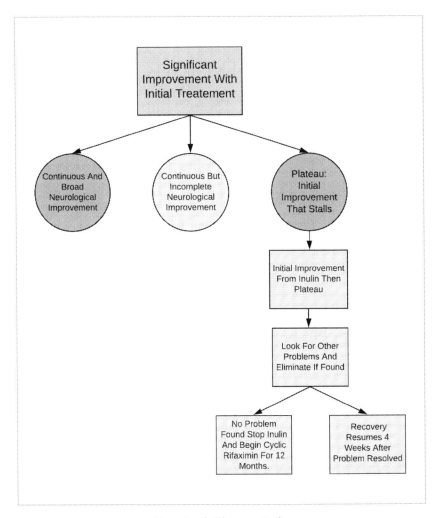

Managing the Plateau on Inulin

I have mentioned before I am are not certain why inulin failure occurs, but I speculate that it is because a different species of bacteria that is unresponsive to the prebiotic effects of inulin now inhabits the small intestine.

Remember, the intestinal microbiota (the collection of all intestinal bacteria) is composed of a thousand or more different species, each with potentially different responses to the prebiotic effects of inulin.

A child's blend of intestinal bacteria naturally changes as children approach ten years of age and older. It is quite possible that young children with bacterial overgrowth of the small intestine tend to initially be overgrown with a species of bacteria that positively respond to the prebiotic effects of inulin.

Given enough time or some other unknown factor, a different bacterium that is not controlled by inulin may begin growing in the small intestine. This bacterium can also trigger the leakage of pro-inflammatory cytokines that flow into the brain which causes the child's recovery to plateau.

In adults, 75% of cases of bacterial overgrowth occurs with only a single species of colonic bacteria overgrowing within the small intestine. In approximately 24% of cases, small intestine bacterial overgrowth occurs with the presence of just two colonic species. The overgrowth species can vary from person to person. Similar studies have not yet been performed in children.

Now, imagine that the single bacterial species involved in overgrowth in a young child is inhibited by the prebiotic effects of inulin. We will refer to this species as bacteria type A.

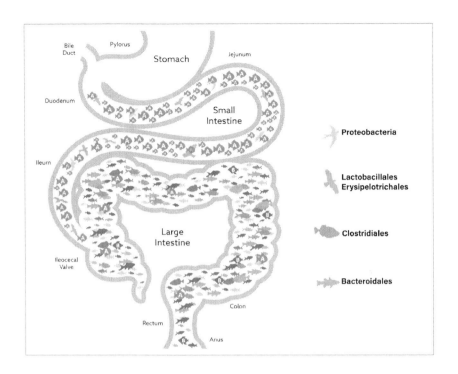

Overgrowth with Bacteria Type A that are Sensitive to the Effects of Inulin

Because bacteria A is inhibited by the addition of inulin it adequately controls the overgrowth allowing neurological recovery to occur. However, there remain a thousand other species within the colon, many of which are not controlled by inulin.

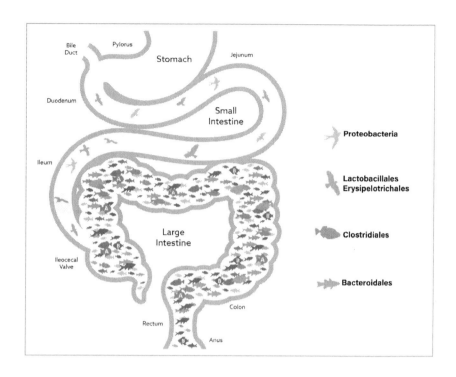

Bile Duct

Pylorus

Stomach

Jejunum

Duodenum

Small Intestine

Proteobacteria

Ileum

Lactobacillales
Erysipelotrichales

Large Intestine

Clostridiales

Ileocecal Valve

Bacteroidales

Colon

Rectum

Anus

Intestinal Bacteria Rebalanced Because of Inulin

Over time as the child's intestine bacteria naturally evolves, an inulin-resistant species (species B) may eventually migrate its way into the small intestine and grow in an uncontrolled manner and become the new form of bacterial overgrowth that is now resistant to inulin.

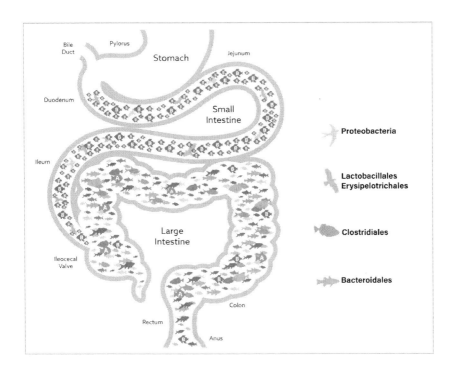

Bile Duct
Pylorus
Stomach
Jejunum
Duodenum
Small Intestine
Ileum
Large Intestine
Ileocecal Valve
Colon
Rectum
Anus

Proteobacteria

Lactobacillales
Erysipelotrichales

Clostridiales

Bacteroidales

Overgrowth with Bacteria Type B that are Resistant
to the Effects of Inulin

The inulin-resistant overgrowth will once again trigger the same series of events that leads to excessive inflammation and halting prior recovery resulting in further developmental delay and cumulative brain injuries.

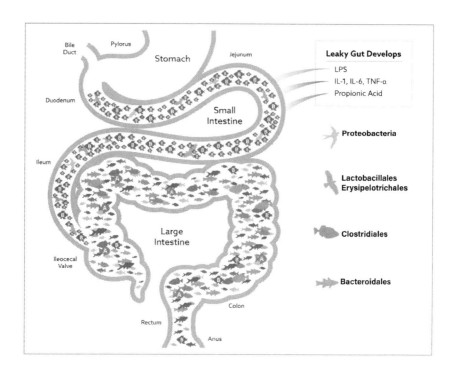

Leakage of Inflammatory Cytokines can
Flow into the Nervous System and Inhibit Recovery

If I suspect my patient is experiencing inulin failure and has hit the plateau, I believe the best treatment course at this point is to discontinue inulin and treat the child with a ten-day course of rifaximin. Inulin is not restarted after treatment with rifaximin since its beneficial effects have proven inadequate to control overgrowth.

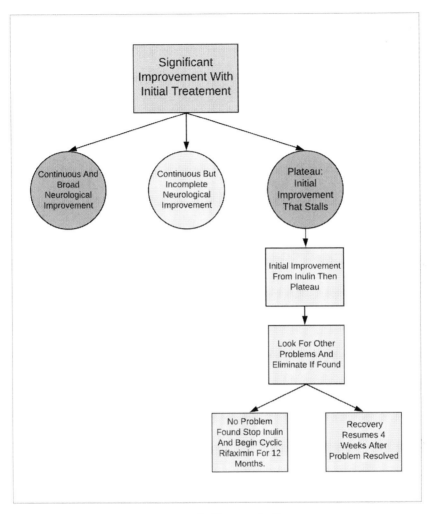

Managing the Plateau on Inulin

When a child has obvious symptoms that improve with rifaximin but obviously return with bacterial relapse (poor eye contact, decreased responsiveness, eczema, aggression, or diarrhea), intermittent rifaximin therapy on an as needed basis seems to work well as a rifaximin strategy.

Rifaximin is a unique antibiotic and some researchers have suggested that it be put into a new medication category called "eubiotic." This term is suggested because rifaximin has a neutral effect on the gut microbiome, unlike most other antibiotics.

Unlike other common antibiotics, rifaximin does not lower intestinal bacterial biodiversity, and the development of long-term bacterial resistance to rifaximin is rare even with continuous, daily dosing over a year or more. And because rifaximin is not absorbed into the bloodstream, it is difficult for rifaximin to abnormally interact with other medications, irritate other organs such as the liver, or cause systemic side effects.

If resistance to rifaximin does occur, I have my patient simply stop rifaximin for a few weeks which results in the disappearance of resistant strains of bacteria. If a rifaximin resistant strain develops while taking a 10-day course of rifaximin, the resistant strain would predictably disappear in the 20 days between each cycle.

Managing a Plateau in a Child Previously Treated with Rifaximin

In a patient previously treated with a single round of rifaximin whose recovery has been halted, the same approach of looking for factors that might interrupt or trigger a relapse of bacterial overgrowth is required. Note that the list of factors able to trigger relapse after the use of rifaximin is longer than the list of factors able to trigger temporary relapse while using inulin.

Factors That Interrupt Recovery After Rifaximin Use

- Physical or Emotional Trauma
- General Anesthesia
- Treatment with Antibiotic
- New Supplement Added
- New Probiotic Added
- Chronic Infection
- Abdominal Surgery
- Colonoscopy

If the recovery of a child previously treated with a single round of rifaximin seems to slow or even stop, this plateau in their recovery is due to a relapse of bacterial overgrowth within the small intestine and they will need to be re-treated with rifaximin. This plateau is similar to what can occur with inulin failure.

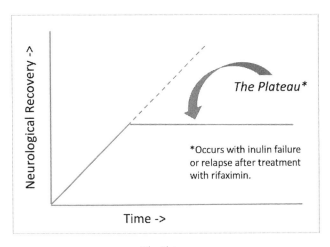

The Plateau

The Plateau

After repeating the second round of rifaximin, the child should begin experiencing neurological renewed improvement about four weeks after completing the rifaximin. Unfortunately, many children seem to relapse within the next month or two after the initial course of rifaximin. Their symptoms of relapse are not very obvious and often can only be determined deductively by the lack of recovery.

Because the rapid relapsing will stop recovery, I generally recommend repeating the ten-day cycle of rifaximin every month on a regular schedule for a minimum of twelve months. I refer to this as "cycling rifaximin." For example, if the first month the child receives the rifaximin on the 5th through the 14th of that month, they will be given rifaximin on the 5th through the 14th of each of the next eleven months.

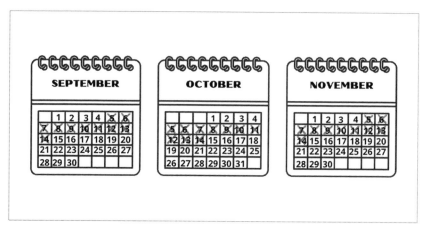

Monthly Cycles of Rifaximin

Often by the end of the twelfth cycle, the child will have experienced significant levels of improvement without interruption. In my current practice, I have several hundred children cycling rifaximin, and it is proving to be an extremely safe and effective approach to maintain a consistent path of recovery.

Many parents are opting to continue monthly cycles of rifaximin even after the initial twelve months to avoid the risk of relapsing and continue their children's recovery.

After twelve months of cyclic rifaximin, some children will have enough recovery of gut motility that their risk of developing bacterial overgrowth again after stopping rifaximin is reduced.

These children can be transitioned to intermittent rifaximin where the repeated courses of rifaximin are based on parental observations that the child has plateaued in their recovery. The only way to determine how rapidly a child might relapse is to simply stop giving rifaximin and see what happens to the child's recovery progress.

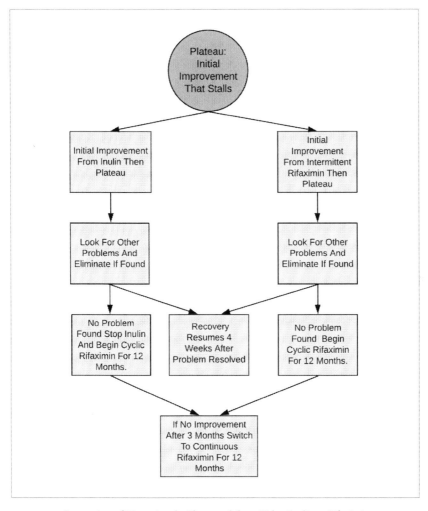

Comparison of Managing the Plateau while on Either Inulin or Rifaximin

Relapse of Bacterial Overgrowth within the Small Intestine

The three major factors known to contribute to small intestine bacterial overgrowth are loss of biodiversity of the gut microbiome, slow intestinal motility, and external factors.

The loss of bacterial species of the gut microbiome has been occurring slowly over many generations as additional damage to gut bacteria from antibiotics, preservatives, pesticides, etc., is passed on from mother to child, and subsequently from female children to their children.

Slow intestinal motility is a well-known predisposing risk factor for bacterial overgrowth and can occur secondarily from autonomic nervous system dysfunction from acute events (acute brain injury or concussion, cumulative brain injury) and medical conditions (chronic inflammatory stress, scleroderma, chronic renal failure).

External factors can trigger bacterial overgrowth as well, and these include medications and supplements (PPI antacids, antibiotics, or probiotics), general anesthesia, medical procedures (gall bladder surgery, appendectomy, hysterectomy, stomach or bowel resection), and acute intestinal infections.

Causes of Recurrent Bacterial Overgrowth

Low Biodiversity
Slow Intestinal Motility
Proton Pump Inhibitors
Use of Antibiotics
Abdominal Surgery
General Anesthesia
Acute Intestinal Infections

The most likely cause of repeated relapse is from slow motility of the intestinal tract due to underlying autonomic dysfunction often from previous brain injuries. The ANS controls the forward propulsion of the intestinal tract if the ANS becomes damaged, the intestinal tracts forward propulsion slows down. The brain injuries can be relatively minor but because of the cumulative brain injury phenomenon, they will build upon each other and have a substantial impact on the child. See chapters fourteen and seventeen for more information on cumulative brain injury.

Rapid relapsing is common in adult patients and they often need to be treated with repeated courses of rifaximin. I have found after three-to-six cycles of rifaximin, their autonomic nervous system function and intestinal motility improve enough that their need for repeated rifaximin slows or stops.

The chronic use of antacids known as proton pump inhibitors (PPIs) are also a frequent cause of relapse of bacterial overgrowth. The flow of stomach acid into the small intestine is an important barrier to the overgrowth of bacteria within the small intestine. PPI antacids result in a profound reduction of stomach acid production and can result in overgrowth of bacterial within the small intestine.

PPIs are often prescribed in children because of severe gastroesophageal reflux and cannot simply be stopped because of the potential damage that might occur to the child's esophagus as well as the pain the child might experience. Since esophageal reflux can cause permanent scarring and narrowing of the esophagus, I strongly recommend not stopping PPI therapy without first consulting the prescribing physician.

Another contributing factor to recurrent bacterial overgrowth is from low biodiversity of intestinal bacterial (low number of intestinal bacterial species). In studies of adults with recurrent *Clostridium difficle* enterocolitis (a form of bacterial overgrowth with a single, toxic bacterial species), the subjects with the lowest biodiversity are most apt to spontaneously relapse or simply not respond to antibiotic therapy whatsoever.

Although the list of precipitating factors for recurrent bacterial overgrowth is small, I expect the list to grow as more and more relapse-triggering environmental factors are identified.

7

INCOMPLETE RECOVERY

Occasionally, I see scenarios where the recovery seems to be partial or incomplete. An example of this might be when despite improvements in comprehension, expressive communication, and socialization the child is having little to no improvements in another neurological aspect such as gross motor skill. Or, it could a child with improvements in speech, socialization, and constipation but their intense hyperactivity and tantrums have not shown any signs of improvement.

If recovery is continuing in some areas but not in others, I recommend the addition of five minutes of transcutaneous vagus nerve stimulation (tVNS) per day. This will reduce the levels of inflammation within the brain further allowing the remaining areas to begin recovering as well.

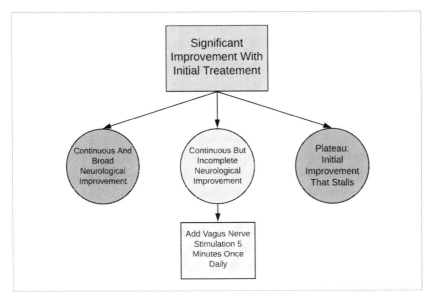

Managing Incomplete Recovery

Vagus nerve stimulation does not increase the speed of recovery but it lowers inflammation further to help encourage all areas of the nervous system to recover.

Often within 6-8 weeks of starting vagus nerve stimulation, the neurological aspects that were lagging behind also start to improve.

In my work with parents and their children, I have seen several charts and diaries logging a child's daily functioning and dosages. While keeping track of dosage changes is important, I recommend charting neurological progress, but *only once a month.* Since neurological recovery is a slow process, all children have "good days and bad days." Charting too frequently might lead to the misinterpretation of the routine ups-and-downs in a child's behavior as a relapse and add to the anxiety of the parents.

Over focusing on behavioral changes that occur in the short term is a common mistake and often leads to unnecessary changes in therapy. Remember, even the behavior of neurotypical children can fluctuate from day-to-day. Having a bad day or bad week is often of no consequence and efforts to determine the causes of each good or bad event will often lead to false conclusions, errors in treatment, and emotional exhaustion for the parent.

Also remember that although two children with autism may have lapsed into autism at the same age and start the protocol at a similar age, they can have very different paths of recovery because they do not necessarily start out with the same level of developmental delay or the same number of injuries. Overgrowth with difference species of bacterial may result in differing levels of inflammation and propionic acid production leading to a greater or lesser degrees of poor eye contact or lack of awareness.

Different brain trauma (physical, emotional, and inflammatory) histories will result in different levels of cumulative brain injury each child is expressing and often manifesting as hyperactivity, anxiety, aggression, gastroesophageal reflux and constipation. Genetic differences between the two children can result in different sensitivities of the brain to chronic inflammation leading to varying degrees of developmental delay (mild, moderate or arrest).

The Addition of Vagus Nerve Stimulation

I will explain the science of vagus nerve stimulation (VNS) at length in chapters ten and eleven but for purposes of understanding it is a treatment element of The Nemechek Protocol® I mention here as well.

Vagus nerve stimulation (VNS) improves recovery by further reducing inflammation within the child's brain, thereby allowing the brain's natural repair, pruning and rejuvenation mechanisms to work more effectively throughout the entire brain.

Stimulation of the vagus nerve can be done by either surgically implanting a device in the chest or by placing an electrode clip to the front and back of a certain areas of the ear called the concha and the tragus. Stimulation through the skin is referred to as transcutaneous VNS (tVNS) and uses such low currents that the child is unable to feel any electrical sensation and only feels the gentle pressure of the clip.

Transcutaneous VNS only needs to be done five minutes per day and can be done while the child is either awake or asleep. VNS has a proven safety record over decades of use for treatment for epilepsy and depression. Although five minutes of VNS per day seems insignificant, it has the potential to lower systemic inflammation for 24-36 hours.

Remember, the ultimate goal of The Nemechek Protocol® is to lower inflammation within the brain enough to allow the nervous system to repair itself.

In summary, tVNS is not required for all children because in my experience many can fully recover from autism and developmental delay without it. If my patient seems to be recovering fully, vagus nerve stimulation is not required and its use will not speed up recovery. If my patient is improving but certain aspects of their neurological impairment are lagging behind, I recommend the addition of tVNS. And finally, in my experience, children thirteen years or older will often require vagus nerve stimulation.

8

LITTLE TO NO IMPROVEMENT

Strategies for Managing Inulin Intolerance, No Response to
Inulin or Rifaximin, and Failure of Rifaximin Cycling

As the following graphic illustrates, the initial response to
The Nemechek Protocol® may be intolerable, non-existent
or temporary. Determining which applies to the patient's
scenario helps me guide parents when presenting the information
outlined in this section.

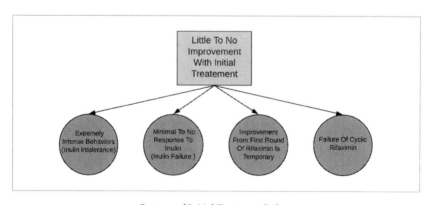

Patterns of Initial Treatment Failure

Managing Inulin Intolerance

Occasionally some children will have a very intense reaction to inulin even at extremely low doses. The most common intense side effects of inulin are increased hyperactivity, anxiety, and maybe even aggression which can sometimes be managed by lowering the dosage of inulin and still maintaining the pace of recovery. Some children will have these reactions even at doses a low as 1/32 tsp. or 1/64 tsp of inulin per day.

In other cases, some parents have mistakenly been increasing the inulin to doses of one-to-two teaspoons per day in hopes of increasing the rate of recovery or of forcing certain aspects such as speech to occur. These extremely high doses of inulin can also trigger the same anxiety, aggression, and hyperactivity in their children.

The anxiety, aggression, and hyperactivity noted by parents are then mistakenly being called a "second awakening" when in fact it is simply what I refer to as inulin intolerance. The reason for such an excessively strong reaction to inulin is unclear but it is clinically consistent with suboptimal brain blood pressure with resulting suboptimal oxygen delivery.

Hyperactivity, increased hunger, and increased thirst are reflexive responses by the brain that often result in improved brain blood pressure and oxygen delivery to the brain.

The anxiety and aggression are symptoms from the release of noradrenaline, the body's natural fight (aggression) or flight (panic, anxiety) hormone. Noradrenaline will increase blood pressure to the brain and alleviate the low oxygen stress but unfortunately causes the fight or flight symptoms.

At this point, I believe the best option is to discontinue inulin completely and treat the patient with a ten-day course of rifaximin. Rebalancing the intestinal bacteria with rifaximin does not result in the same type of adverse response and is equally effective at reducing bacterial overgrowth.

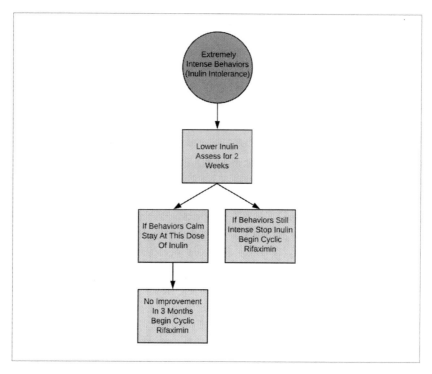

Managing Inulin Intolerance

In my experience, many patients may have a relapse of bacterial over-growth within four-to-eight weeks of the first round of rifaximin. This seems to happen so commonly that when starting rifaximin after inulin failure, I often recommend starting the children on repeated ten-day courses of cyclic rifaximin each month for a minimum of twelve months.

For example, if the child receives the first round of rifaximin on April 4th through the 13th, they will receive another round on May 4th through the 13th, June 4th through the 13th, and so on.

Cyclic rifaximin dosing has been a breakthrough in establishing a consistent path of recovery for my patients with autism and developmental delay.

The improvements seen by the twelve-month time point are often so impressive that many parents opt to continue cycling rifaximin until which time their child is behaving in a neurotypical fashion.

Minimal to No Response After Initial Treatment with Inulin

The least common response to The Nemechek Protocol® in my patients is that no significant improvement in autistic or developmental issues is observed after the first three to six months on the protocol.

Children initially failing the protocol may continue to have some small improvements because of other therapeutic efforts (for instance speech or occupational therapy) but there will be no significant increase in the pace of recovery.

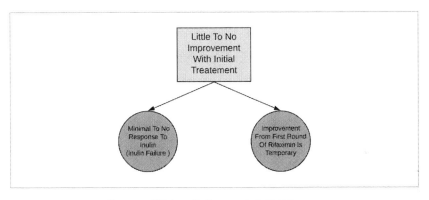

Patterns of Little to No Response to Initial Therapy

A word of caution before deciding that that initial use of inulin did not work. Many parents tend to over-focus on wanting to see improvements in speech or socialization initially and will overlook improvements that are occurring in receptive communication, fine or gross motor skills, anger control, or sensory-seeking behaviors.

The ability to speak is extremely complex and does not start to recover until complex levels of receptive communication skills have developed. Likewise, learning to socialize with unfamiliar children often only occurs after learning to socialize with the child's parents, siblings, and unfamiliar adults.

The intense desire to see their child communicate normally and play with other children is quite natural for the parents, but unfortunately these are some of the most complicated behaviors to master and often occur later or last, not sooner, in the recovery process.

If there has been no substantial increase in recovery despite taking inulin and there is no interference from probiotics, antibiotics, supplements, or a chronic illness, then the child has experienced inulin failure. I recommend treatment with rifaximin. Inulin is not restarted after I treat them with rifaximin.

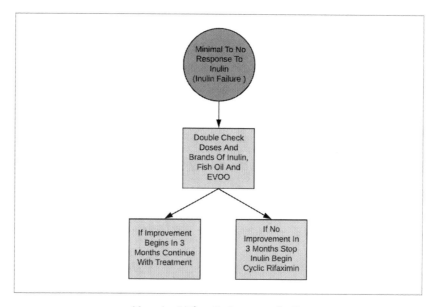

Managing Little to No Response to Inulin

Minimal to No Response after Initial Treatment with Rifaximin

Sometimes after a patient is treated with rifaximin there is no improvement, or the child seems to relapse within just a few days or weeks. These children are experiencing a rapid relapse of bacterial overgrowth within the small intestine. These rapid relapses are most likely due to slow intestinal motility from underlying autonomic dysfunction (see chapters ten and fourteen).

My most effective approach in this scenario is to begin cycling rifaximin with monthly ten-day courses of rifaximin for a minimum of twelve months. The point of cycling is to keep the bacterial overgrowth suppressed enough to allow the child's nervous system to continue recovering.

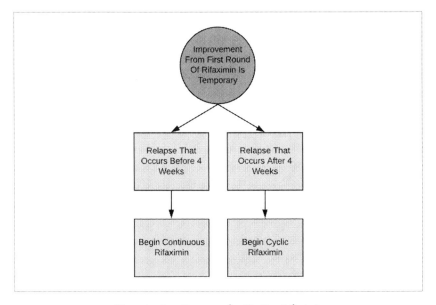

Managing Poor Response after Starting Rifaximin

Managing Failure of Rifaximin Cycling

Even with monthly rifaximin some patients still will not show evidence of recovery and this is because they are relapsing even before the next course of rifaximin has begun.

If a patient is not showing any improvement after three months of rifaximin, I start these patients on non-stop, twice daily, continuous rifaximin along with five minutes of daily vagus nerve stimulation.

The primary reason the children are relapsing rapidly is because of slow intestinal motility often from autonomic nervous system damage. It is my hope that the addition of vagus nerve stimulation in the patient will help insure their intestinal motility can improve to a degree that continuous rifaximin can ultimately be discontinued.

My first cases requiring continuous rifaximin involved extremely violent, older children (sixteen-to-twenty years of age) with autism. These patients would have a significant decrease in their violent tendencies while on rifaximin but then would relapse within a few days of finishing the course of ten days. I found increasing the course of rifaximin to fourteen or twenty-one days was no more effective in preventing the relapses.

After starting on the continuous, twice daily rifaximin, their violent behavior declined and did not increase again. Over time, their behavior improved so much that the dosages and number of psychiatric medications they had been described were reduced and often discontinued. In several such cases, the parents have opted to stay on the continuous rifaximin fearful that the violent relapses might occur once again.

After twelve months of continuous therapy, I recommend reducing rifaximin therapy to the monthly cycle of ten-day courses. If recovery stops again because of relapsing bacteria, I restart continuous therapy again for the patient for another 6 months and then try reducing to monthly cycles again. With more time, my hope is the monthly cycles of rifaximin might also be discontinued with rifaximin only needing to be used occasionally.

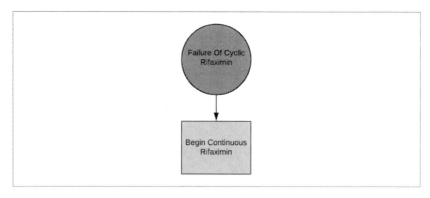

Managing Failure of Cyclic Rifaximin

Daily, continuous rifaximin has been safely used for almost thirty years in patients with advanced cirrhosis of the liver who develop hepatic encephalopathy. Patients with hepatic encephalopathy are placed on twice daily rifaximin continuously to prevent dangerous ammonia production. Studies indicate the continuous use of rifaximin does not lower the bacterial biodiversity within the gut microbiome.

Although bacterial resistance to rifaximin occurs very rarely, the resistance quickly disappears after discontinuing rifaximin for only a few weeks. The rifaximin can then be restarted with the same positive effect.

In review, after initiating the protocol with the appropriate dose of fish oil and olive oil and starting to balance the intestinal tract with either inulin or rifaximin, I observe and make note of the degree of recovery that occurs in the following three months.

If there is a significant suppression of bacterial overgrowth, the child will experience notable improvements. If most, but not all, aspects of their neurological problems are improving, I believe adding adding five minutes of daily vagus nerve stimulation is necessary to encourage all developmental issues to begin recovering.

If there is only a temporary improvement, minimal improvement, or treatment with inulin causes too many side effects, the flow charts presented earlier in this chapter illustrate will help you understand how I determine the dosing of rifaximin in single, cyclic or continuous dosing strategies to move my patients forward in the recovery process.

9

WHEN AND IF TO STOP THE NEMECHEKPROTOCOL

After a few years on The Nemechek Protocol®, many children will recover enough to reach a neurotypical state. The next obvious question is which components of the protocol can be stopped and which components might need to be continued?

In my adult patients recovering on the protocol, most will experience a partial relapse of their prior cumulative brain injuries if they stop or decrease any of the components (fish oil, olive oil, vagus stimulation, and maintaining a balanced intestinal tract).

I think recurrence in cumulative brain injury will similarly apply to the children treated with the protocol with a major exception that involves a special white blood cell in the brain called a primed microglia. I will discuss primed microglia further on in this chapter.

The brain learns to speak, socialize and process sensory inputs by pruning away neurons. Improvement in developmental function occur as excessive neurons within the brain are pruned away. Therefore, a relapse would require an increase in the overall number of neurons and there is no medical evidence that once pruned away, more neurons would accumulate with an increase in inflammatory stress.

But why do the cumulative brain injuries recur after stopping the protocol? Understandably, many people mistakenly assume that recovery from a brain injury is like healing a broken bone. Once the injury is healed you no longer need the treatment or the arm cast in the case of a fracture.

A major difference between a chronic brain injury and a forearm fracture is that a brain injury has become chronic because of the formation of a permanent population of harmful cells called primed microglia.

Microglia are a population of special white blood cells that only live in the brain and they are involved in the normal pruning of neurons during the developmental process and the repair of neurons after injury. Unfortunately, bacterial overgrowth can alter the behavior of microglia that will lead to a recurrence of cumulative brain injury if the protocol is stopped.

Primed Microglia Cause Relapses from Chronic Brain Injury

Primed microglia are formed after lipopolysaccharide (LPS) from bacterial overgrowth (SIBO, small intestine bacterial overgrowth) leaks into the bloodstream and eventually migrates to the brain and encounters healthy microglia.

LPS transforms healthy microglia into harmful inflammatory microglia, which are referred to as primed microglia. They are also referred to as primed M1-microglia.

Unlike healthy microglia that are regularly replaced with new normal functioning microglia every few months, primed microglia never die and constantly leak inflammatory cytokines into their surrounding area.

The inflammatory stress these inflammatory cytokines create prevents the neurons in the same area from being repaired and will magnify the damage in future injuries.

The protocol's combination of vagus nerve stimulation, olive oil, and high concentrations of the omega-3 fatty acid DHA help control the damaging inflammatory behavior of primed microglia through a process called phenotypic shifting.

As long as these ingredients are given consistently in the correct dosages, the primed microglia change their behavior and start helping with the repair process. Maintaining the primed microglia in a helpful, repairing mode (often referred to M2-microglia) also reduces their production of damaging inflammatory cytokines and improves the ability of nearby neurons to recover.

At present, there is no known treatment to eradicate primed microglia and therefore they need to be controlled over the long term in order to maintain one's recovery from a previously unresolved brain injury. There is growing evidence in animal studies that the elimination of primed microglia may one day be possible. Most of this work is looking at chemical compounds known as CSFR1-inhibitors.

Vagus nerve stimulation, fish oil, and olive oil will all need to be continued for the long term until other methods of eliminating primed microglia are found.

There is another reason why some of The Nemechek Protocol® ingredients should not be stopped. Since there is no effort by the food industry to remove the excessive amounts of inflammatory linoleic acid from the food supply, the need for olive oil in our diet to protect us from these omega-6 fatty acids will remain.

Similarly, the lack of anti-inflammatory omega-3 fatty acids in the food supply necessitates long-term supplementation with omega-3 fatty acids sourced from fish and other marine sources to assist our cells in regulating inflammation.

As the stocks of fish in the oceans become more and more depleted, other forms of omega-3 fatty acids may need to be produced from algae or other recombinant technologies.

On the distant horizon is the hope of pharmaceutical therapies that can rid the nervous system of these permanently damaging primed microglia. A class of agents known as CsfıR inhibitors are showing promising results are permanently halting the chronic inflammatory damage from primed microglia in preclinical animal trials.

Potential Relapses in Children Differ from Adults

The situation is not so straightforward in children because they have recovered from both cumulative brain injuries and developmental delay. Although both require a normal microglial function to recover, there is a unique difference in children's recovery that prevents relapses in developmental delay.

Children who have recovered from cumulative brain injuries often relapse similarly as adults. The most common symptoms associated with cumulative brain injuries that might return in children include: hyperactivity, toe-walking, anxiety, OCD, fearfulness, aggressiveness, rage events, flight events, increased hunger and thirst, poor focus and concentration including ADD and ADHD, constipation, abdominal cramping and heartburn or reflux, and insomnia.

Relapsing from developmental delay is a different matter. In order for a child realize their developmental milestones, a child needs to prune away fifty per cent of the neurons within their brain. Synaptic pruning is the brain's way of removing unnecessary connections that are not needed which strengthens the ones that are required to mature and lock in a new developmental skill.

Once pruned away, these neurons are gone forever, never to return. Developmental delays occur when there is incomplete or slowed pruning of the neurons of the brain.

The Nemechek Protocol® resolves developmental delays by allowing the microglia to begin finally prune away the excessive neurons and this leads to developmental gains. There are truly fewer neurons when your child has recovered developmentally than when they were delayed.

For this reason, I do not believe true relapses after recovery from a developmental delay are possible. These children do not "unlearn" the developmental milestones they have reached. Since recovery from developmental delay involves permanently removing neurons, relapse from developmental delay cannot occur because the neurons would need to be added back, and this is not believed to be possible.

I have heard many times that a child has "lost" this or that developmental function, and I understand the comment from the parent's perspective. In truth, the prior gains are still present, but simply not visible to the parent and not accessible to the child often because of the child's increased anxiety, worsened focus, and toxic effects of propionic acid.

This phenomenon is no different from an adult who cannot think or speak clearly when in front of an audience (which is akin to stage fright). With more practice at public speaking, the adult is finally able to speak well even when feeling anxious or under stress. Similarly, a child with continued recovery will also be able to use more complex speech even when feeling anxious.

Long Term Challenges of Maintaining a Healthy Balance of Intestinal Bacteria

Reversal and prevention of bacterial overgrowth in the small intestine (SIBO) is required for recovery from developmental delay and brain injuries in children. If SIBO returns, the inflammatory stress from this is so great all recovery comes to a halt. After recovery has been achieved, maintaining a healthy balance of intestinal bacteria in children (and adults) can be a challenge.

The three known factors involved in relapses of bacterial overgrowth of the small intestine are the slowing of intestinal motility, intermittent disruption of the intestinal bacteria by infections or medications, and low intestinal biodiversity.

Slowed Intestinal Motility

Spontaneous relapses from slowed intestinal motility are due to underlying autonomic dysfunction from cumulative brain injury. With time on the protocol, the autonomic dysfunction leading to relapses in this manner will substantially improve during the course of the child's recovery. Slow intestinal motility is the most frequent cause of relapsing bacterial overgrowth in children and adults.

Disruption of Intestinal Balance

Intermittent disruption of bacterial balance often cannot be avoided because it can be triggered by common infections (viral and bacterial gastroenteritis) or the use of necessary medications (antibiotics, chemotherapy, proton pump inhibitors). Regrettably, this source of relapse will continue until medical science discovers how to treat infections without gut damaging antibiotics or manage severe acid reflux without proton pump inhibitors.

Low Intestinal Biodiversity

Low biodiversity is known to predispose people to spontaneous bacterial overgrowth only when the level of biodiversity is severely depleted. In studies of *Clostridium difficle* enterocolitis, frequent relapses of bacterial overgrowth occur when the individual's intestinal gut microbiome has been depleted to about 70% of normal bacterial species.

Treatment of this requires a fecal microbiota transplant (FMT), commonly referred to as a human stool transplant. Most studies of FMT in patients with higher levels of biodiversity (>80%) seem to have little to no benefit. The majority of the biodiversity of studies in children with autism or developmental problems do not indicate severe depletion of biodiversity. Because of this, I do not recommend FMT. In addition, I have been involved in the care of many children who have received FMT but still had frequent relapses of bacterial overgrowth, so FMT was of no benefit to them in their neurological recovery.

Long Term Inulin to Prevent Bacterial Relapses

As a child ages, there is an increasing tendency that inulin will no longer be able to control bacterial overgrowth and by twenty years of age, inulin is ineffective in controlling bacterial overgrowth enough to obtain a substantial degree of brain recovery.

The reason for this is not precisely understood but most likely has to do with the tendency of overgrowth in adults being from a bacterial species whose growth is not suppressed by inulin.

The long-term use of daily inulin in children is very safe, inexpensive, and controls SIBO as long as it remains effective. Eventually, as the child ages, the inulin will likely fail, and bacterial overgrowth will return.

At this point, the child will need to be transitioned to intermittent courses of rifaximin to control any symptoms that occur from bacterial overgrowth.

Managing Bacterial Overgrowth with Rifaximin

Many children under my care today receive monthly courses of rifaximin (during cyclic rifaximin) in order to prevent relapsing of bacterial overgrowth. A smaller proportion of children are receiving rifaximin non-stop without any intermittent breaks in treatment ("continuous rifaximin") and an even smaller proportion are receiving intermittent rifaximin only as needed for recognizable relapses.

Over time, from treating neurotypical adult patients, I have learned that their intestinal motility will improve, and the relapses of bacterial overgrowth become less and less frequent so we can taper off rifaximin. This seems to hold true for children as well.

My overall approach is to reduce the frequency of rifaximin in children as they recover. If a child was only able to experience recovery with continuous, non-stop rifaximin therapy because they were relapsing very quickly, I found it will take a minimum of twelve months of rifaximin before intestinal motility recovers enough that the rifaximin can be changed from continuous to the less intense schedule of monthly cycles of rifaximin.

After another six-to-twelve months on cyclic rifaximin, there is a good chance the child can be tapered off rifaximin to just intermittent rifaximin.

And likewise, if a child's recovery improved with cyclic rifaximin, I recommend a minimum of twelve monthly cycles before trying to shift to intermittent rifaximin.

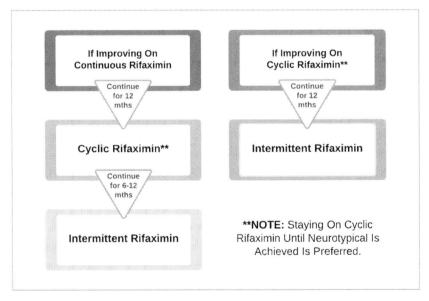

Considerations on the Reduction of Rifaximin Dosing

Many parents are opting to use rifaximin for even longer than twelve months in order to prevent any delays in recovery from the inevitable relapses, and as of this writing, I care for some older children with autism who have been treated with both cyclic and continuous rifaximin for up to three years without complication.

PART III

VAGUS NERVE STIMULATION

10

THE USE OF VAGUS NERVE STIMULATION IN CHILDHOOD DISORDERS

This chapter will explain in greater detail vagus nerve stimulation (VNS) and the role it plays in The Nemechek Protocol®.

The vagus nerve is one of the most important nerves in the body. Commonly referred to as the tenth cranial nerve, it runs down either side of the neck, fusing together below the breastbone to form a single trunk and branching out to the body's organs and blood vessels.

Generally, nerves are often visualized as a strand of biological wire that carries electrical impulses from the brain to different areas of the body. However, the vagus nerve is much, much more complex.

The vagus nerve consists of approximately 60,000 different nerve fibers bundled together like a fiber-optic cable. These nerves transmit information and instructions as electrical impulses, and these signals travel from the body up to the brain and from the brain down to the body.

About 80% of the information and instructions carried by the vagus nerve travels from the body upwards into the brain in what is referred to as afferent fibers. The remaining 20% of information on the vagus nerve travels downward from the brain to the body to help regulate inflammation and other organ functions. These downward brain to the body fibers are called efferent fibers.

The autonomic nervous system (ANS) has two branches or controlling arms: the parasympathetic and the sympathetic nervous systems. These branches allow the brain to regulate every single aspect of the body's function.

The vagus nerve is the main conduit of signals from the parasympathetic branch. The sympathetic branch runs through the spinal cord and sends out smaller branches between each pair of vertebrae. Signals carried by the sympathetic branch travel both upwards and downwards.

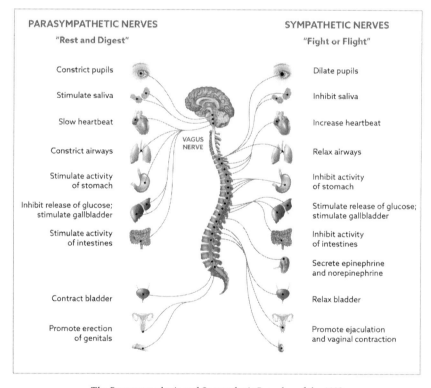

The Parasympathetic and Sympathetic Branches of the ANS

Through parasympathetic pathways of the vagus nerve, the brain "listens" to how the organs are functioning and monitors the body's level of stress (infection, injury, or toxins) as a variety of signals are sent upwards.

Signals from the vagus nerve are interpreted by a variety of different regions of the brain. The brain interprets the signals and responds by sending signals downward through the efferent fibers of the vagus nerve, the sympathetic fibers in the spinal cord, and by releasing hormones from the pituitary glands.

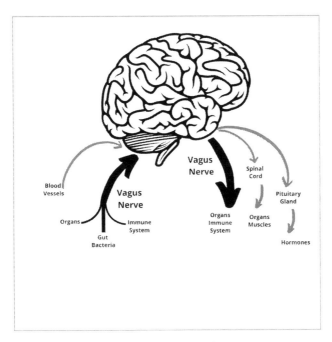

Flow of Signals To and From the Brain

This circular pattern of "listening" through the vagus nerve and then "responding" through the vagus nerve, spinal cord, and hormones is how the brain regulates the body's organs when things are functioning normally when there is a dangerous threat in the area, or if the body is suffering from an infection or an injury.

The Beginnings of Vagus Nerve Stimulation

Back in the 1990s, research suggested that stimulation of the vagus nerve might be a useful approach to control seizures. Researchers developed an implantable vagus nerve stimulating device that is similar to a pacemaker used to increase the heart rate of an ailing heart.

When used for vagus nerve stimulation, the wires are wrapped around the vagus nerve and the electrical impulses stimulate the vagus nerve instead of the heart. These devices send pulsations of electricity and stimulate the vagus nerve 24 hours per day. Vagus nerve stimulators have astonishing remission rates of 50-75% per year for treatment-resistant epilepsy and depression.

Stimulating the Vagus Nerve without Requiring Surgery

A breakthrough in the pursuit of controlling chronic inflammation with vagus stimulation is the ability to use vagus stimulation to control inflammation without requiring a surgically implanted device.

As the vagus nerve runs from the brain down into the neck, a branch from the vagus nerve called the *auricular* branch (auricular is the Latin word for ear) extends out to the center of the ear in regions of the ear referred to as the concha and tragus.

The vagus nerve can be externally stimulated by directly placing a very mild and imperceptible electrical current directly on the skin in these areas.

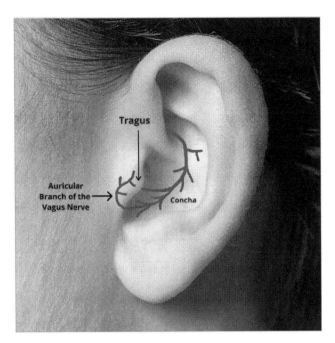

Auricular Branch of the Vagus Nerve

This method is referred to as transcutaneous (meaning across the skin) vagus nerve stimulation or tVNS. Five minutes of tVNS has been shown to be highly effective in lowering systemic inflammation throughout the body for over twenty-four hours.

Avoiding surgery eliminates the risk of surgery-related infections, complications from anesthesia, and dramatically reduces the cost of VNS. TVNS brings the positive health benefits of the treatment into the reach of individuals affected by chronic inflammatory disorders.

Modern Vagus Nerve Stimulation

In the last twenty years, over 120,000 vagus nerve stimulators have been successfully implanted in the United States for epilepsy and depression. In addition to the remarkable improvement in controlling these disorders, vagus nerve stimulation has been found to be a powerful method to suppress unhealthy levels of chronic inflammation.

Chronic inflammation is now understood to be the primary cause of a wide variety of common medical conditions. Inflammation causes illness by either turning on or turning off genes associated with diseases such as diabetes mellitus, cancer, and autoimmune disorders.

Inflammation causes direct damage to tissue and is an important factor in the development of strokes, heart attacks, nerve damage (neuropathy), and chronic pain from fibromyalgia, arthritis, fasciitis, tendonitis, and bursitis.

Lastly, chronic inflammation within the central nervous system impairs the nervous system's natural repair mechanisms and is primarily responsible for the development of Alzheimer's dementia, Parkinson's ataxia, chronic depression, schizophrenia, PTSD, and bipolar disorder.

General Effects of Chronic Inflammation
- Trigger Genetically Associated Disease State
- Direct Damage to Tissue within the Body
- Impairment of Tissue Repair Mechanisms
- Suppression of Stem Cell Function
- Impairment of Immune Function

In children, chronic inflammation impairs the brain's ability to properly prune neurons, which is required for normal development and leads to developmental issues such as sensory impairment, apraxia, and communication problems.

Inflammation also prevents a child's brain from naturally repairing itself after an injury in a process I refer to as cumulative brain injury.

As investigations into the chronic inflammatory model of disease continue to develop, our understanding of the many ways chronic inflammation can negatively affect the health of a child continues to grow.

Specific Effects of Chronic Inflammation on Children
- Developmental Impairment
- Autism Spectrum Disorders
- Intellectual, Communication Disorders
- Visual Impairment
- Sensory Perception Disorder
- Low Muscle Tone
- Focus and Concentration Issues
- Hyperactivity
- Headaches, Functional Abdominal Pain
- Aggression and Self Injurious Behavior
- Constipation, Bloating and Heartburn
- Chronic Depression, Bipolar Disorder, Anxiety
- Schizophrenia
- Epilepsy
- Growth Impairment
- Chronic or Recurrent Joint or Muscle Pain

Given the wide variety of harmful effects that chronic inflammation has on the human body, vagus nerve stimulation's ability to suppress inflammation is being tested in a variety of conditions other than epilepsy and chronic depression with generally positive results.

In my experience with children, tVNS greatly improves the ability of all areas of the central nervous system to develop properly and improves the brain's ability to recovery from cumulative brain injury.

11

WHEN TO ADD THE VAGUS NERVE STIMULATION

After balancing the intestinal bacteria with either inulin or rifaximin and initiating the proper doses of fish oil and olive oil as described in The Nemechek Protocol®, the next step is to monitor the child's recovery over the following three to six months. I will monitor the patient to determine if all aspects of the child's neurological impairments are moving forward towards recovery.

Over this three to six month period, many of the children under my care will begin to experience improved rates of recovery from developmental delay and cumulative brain injury effects.

All potential aspects of neurological recovery should be monitored in order to assess the effect of the protocol. Items to track include speech, sensory, attention/focus, meaningful play, socialization, aggression, self-injurious behaviors (SIBs), motor skills/tone, intestinal function, and symptoms of low brain blood pressure.

Items to Monitor to Determine Recovery
Speech
Sensory
Socialization
Attention/Focus
Meaningful Play
Aggression/SIBs
Motor Skills/Tone
Intestinal Function
Receptive Communication
Expressive Communication
Symptoms of Low Brain Blood Pressure

Usually, all aspects of development, function, and behavior will steadily improve but occasionally, a child might have one or two areas that do not seem to be improving at all.

For instance, a child might experience great improvements in emotional control, motor function, improvement in sleep, and intestinal function but expressive language and socialization do not seem to be improving after several months.

If, after being on the proper doses of fish oil, olive oil, and either inulin or rifaximin my patient has a few areas that do not seem to be improving, then I believe the child may benefit from the addition of VNS.

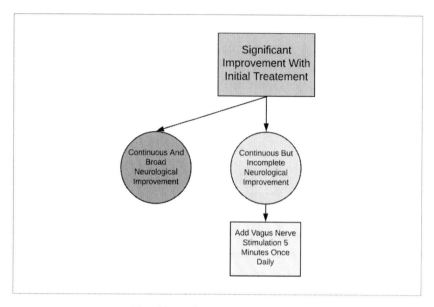

The Addition of Vagus Nerve Stimulation

Transcutaneous VNS assists all developmental areas to recover through its combined effect on suppressing the negative effects of inflammation on neuronal pruning and repair as well as its ability to expand neural networks.

I commonly recommend the use of tVNS in young patients four years and older who are demonstrating incomplete neurological recovery of any sort. Children under four seem to have a much greater chance of recovery without tVNS but they may also be candidates for tVNS if showing signs of incomplete recovery.

Benefits of Vagus Nerve Stimulation in Non-Developmental Conditions

There are several other areas that tVNS may help patients that are not directly related to traditional developmental delay. For instance, vagus nerve stimulation can improve some genetically triggered illnesses, tinnitus, post-concussion syndrome, spinal cord injury, schizophrenia, and cerebral palsy.

<u>Other Potential Benefits of Vagus Nerve Stimulation</u>
Schizophrenia
Cerebral Palsy
Post-Concussion Syndrome
Reduction or Elimination of Tinnitus
Stroke and Spinal Cord Injury

A growing number of studies in adults are even evaluating VNS as a method to improve recovery after ischemic and thrombotic strokes as well as traumatic spinal cord injuries.

Since cerebral palsy is related to brain cell damage from the lack of oxygen, the same benefits seen in stroke and spinal cord injury recovery and cerebral palsy as well. In my private practice, I have seen some rather amazing improvements in children with cerebral palsy.

Finally, the most intriguing but least studied effect of VNS is on genetic remission in chronic inflammatory disorders. Some genes are activated or de-activated by increasing levels of inflammatory stress leading to altered cellular function and triggering what is outwardly diagnosed as a particular disease.

Examples such as diabetes mellitus type 2, rheumatoid arthritis, and many common cancers (breast colon, prostate, brain) are believed to be activated by chronic inflammation.

In about 10% of children who appear on the autism spectrum, the presence of an abnormal gene is detected. The parent is told their child is "at-risk" for developing a particular disease, including autism, associated with the gene. It is important to emphasize that the child will only develop the illness if the identified gene is turned on or activated which is often caused by inflammation.

Furthermore, animal studies suggest that if inflammation is lowered enough, the previously active disease-causing genes can be shut off, resulting in a genetic remission.

I have witnessed this several times in adults with Hashimoto's thyroiditis and Crohn's disease, and I think that genetic remission might be responsible for the recoveries I have witnessed in some children with a variety of genetic abnormalities known to be associated with autism.

Use of Vagus Nerve Stimulation for Other Inflammatory Conditions

As I have been discussing, the health of children and adults is negatively affected by the chronic presence of inflammatory chemicals referred to as pro-inflammatory cytokines. Throughout the world, these chemicals are rising as people age in a process often referred to as inflamm-aging.

Released by white blood cells, inflammatory cytokines circulate in the bloodstream and encounter every cell of the body. The cytokines trigger the activation of molecules such as HMGB-1 and NF-kB which are ultimately responsible for turning on the genes responsible for common diseases like insulin resistance (diabetes), most cancers, and autoimmune disorders such as rheumatoid arthritis and Crohn's disease.

Chronically elevated pro-inflammatory cytokines also cause direct damage to the tissue resulting in chronic pain syndromes, nerve damage (neuropathy), strokes and heart attacks. The chronic production of these cytokines impairs the functioning of stem cell function and other natural repair mechanisms.

In children, chronic inflammation is responsible for inflammatory bowel disease (Crohn's and ulcerative colitis), triggering the genes responsible for other autoimmune disorders such as juvenile arthritis or type 1 diabetes mellitus. Inflammation also causes chronic joint and muscle pain (arthritis), worsens inflammatory skin conditions such as eczema and psoriasis, increases the frequency of epileptic seizures, and can damage peripheral nerves leading to neuropathy.

Utilizing transcutaneous vagus nerve stimulation (tVNS) can significantly reduce inflammation and thus improve these genetically driven disorders. Considering how safe and well-tolerated tVNS is in children, this component of The Nemechek Protocol® provides an opportunity to improve and potentially reverse genetically linked childhood illnesses.

Other Non-Neurological Benefits of Vagus Nerve Simulation
Improved Intestinal Motility
Improved Tolerance of Dietary Gluten
Reduction of Chronic Inflammatory Pain
Improved Control of Autoimmune Disorders

Because of its ability to lower inflammation even further I routinely recommend the addition of tVNS in any child with autism or developmental delay who is experiencing an incomplete recovery using my protocol, is requiring continuous rifaximin to control bacterial overgrowth, or is requiring the use of prescription medications to control behavior or enhance focus and attention.

Other indications of tVNS in children might include an uncontrolled inflammatory or autoimmune disorder, as well as poorly controlled epilepsy.

Expansion of Neural Networks

Another benefit of tVNS results from its ability to help the brain re-establish and expand neural pathways known as neural networks.

The brain functions by sending signals from one area of the brain to another. The concept of a single thought or function between two areas of the brain does not occur through a single linear pathway.

Communication pathways in the brain occur simultaneously through a collection of neurons known as a neural network.

Furthermore, the more neurons that are engaged to achieve the desired function within a particular neural network, the brain's ability to carry out the desired command or instruction becomes more effective.

When a person practices playing a certain musical score over and over on the piano, the neural networks required to read the music and move their fingers appropriately on the keyboard expands. The expansion of the neural network occurs as more and more neurons are crowdsourced to perform a collection of tasks that allows the individual's piano-playing skill to improve.

Likewise, if they cease practicing that particular piece of music, their neural network for that piece of music and for playing the piano in general will shrink, and their performance will worsen in direct proportion of the reduction of that neural network.

Transcutaneous VNS can increase the brain's ability to build and expand these neural networks in a process referred to as cortical plasticity.

Electrical Dosing and Failures After Vagus Nerve Stimulation

The initiation of tVNS to The Nemechek Protocol® jump starts a new pattern of neurological recovery in children and is also a major component of autonomic recovery as applied to neurotypical adults. The purpose of vagus nerve stimulation is to begin substantial recovery in those few areas not yet improving with only fish oil, olive oil, and a balanced intestinal bacterial (inulin or rifaximin).

I have found with my patients that tVNS is often required in patients older than fourteen years of age in order to realize a broader, more complete neurological recovery.

The dosage of electrical stimulation can vary greatly depending on the age of the individual, and the medical condition we are trying to improve. The electrical stimulation parameters vary by intensity, frequency, and timing of cycling of electricity on and off, and total time on device per each twenty-four hour period. The variables for VNS treatments include amperage, band width, frequency (Hz), the cycling pattern (off/on) and the clip's position on the ear.

The vast majority of children and young adults less than thirty years of age will only require five minutes of continuous transcutaneous vagus nerve stimulation per day. At the proper settings, five minutes of tVNS is enough to significantly reduce inflammation throughout the body for at least twenty-four hours.

Five minutes of tVNS has also been shown to cause the unhealthy primed M1-phenotype microglia to change their behavior and begin acting like the healthy M2-microglia that are once again able to prune and repair neurons. In children with autism and developmental disorders including isolated ADD or ADHD, the M1-to-M2 phenotypic shift is essential to obtain a full recovery. More information of shifting between the M1 and M2 phenotypes is found in chapter fourteen.

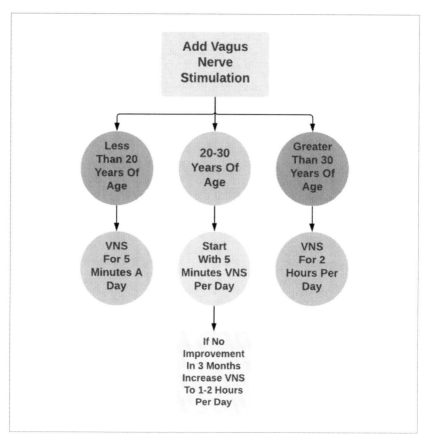

Different Vagus Nerve Stimulation Time Requirements

Between the ages of twenty and thirty, I generally recommend my patients start with five minutes of tVNS per day. When combined with the core aspects of The Nemechek Protocol®, most adults in this age range will begin to experience significant neurological recovery within three months but occasionally there may be some young adults who are an exception.

Often improvements in the neurological deficits begin to improve within six weeks. Although the impact of tVNS on inflammation and microglia behavior occurs immediately, it often takes a few weeks for the improvements to accumulate enough that they become recognizable by the parent or caretaker.

The older the patient is (child -> young adult -> older adult), the slower their rate of neurological recovery may seem. But as a rule, improvement should be recognizable in all patients after one to three months as long as there have not been any substantial interruptions or traumas during this time.

In adults between twenty and thirty years of age, if there is no recognizable improvement after three months of daily five-minute tVNS sessions, I consider the possibility of a relapse of bacterial intestinal imbalance and retreat with rifaximin. Also, I look for interfering supplements and have the patient discontinue them if present.

If neither of these is present and a repeat course of rifaximin fails to restart neurological recovery, then I recommend increasing tVNS to one-to-two hours per day.

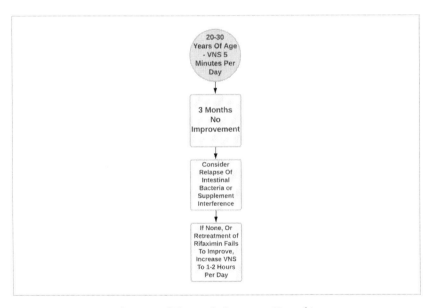

Adjustment of Therapy Patients 20-30 Years of Age

The need to increase tVNS to more than five minutes per day rarely occurs in children under twenty. Within this age group, if there is no significant improvement, it is highly likely that the cause of no neurological improvement is due to a relapse of intestinal bacteria overgrowth rather than the tVNS not being effective.

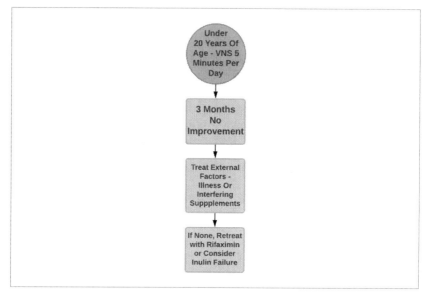

No Adjustment of VNS in Younger Patients is Recommended

This scenario would need to be addressed with another round of rifaximin, initiating cyclic or continuous rifaximin, or if the patient is on inulin I consider it to be inulin failure and I replace inulin with rifaximin. Again, I always look for an external factor such as an intensely stressful situation, supplements, homeopathic remedies, or a probiotic that might be preventing or masking recovery.

There is an exception to the five minutes of tVNS per day rule in children under the age of twenty-five. On occasion, parents will notice that after just five minutes of tVNS, their child may experience a prolonged calming effect that can last for a few hours.

In these cases, I suggest the tVNS be used at least once daily to control inflammation and an additional two to three five-minute increments as needed to control anxiety.

When the tVNS is increased beyond five minutes per day in adults, the electrical current needs to cycle on and off in a particular manner in order to avoid a problem called habituation. Habituation means that the nervous system begins ignoring the electrical stimulating signal as we commonly do with "white noise" or background noises in a room.

After a few years of closely following the recovery patterns of adult patients using tVNS, I developed a highly effective proprietary cycling pattern that prevents habituation but retains its potent ability to reverse cumulative brain injury.

I have found patients over thirty years of age almost universally need two hours of cycling vagus nerve stimulation to recover from cumulative brain injury or to further their recovery from autism and developmental delay. Just as in children, if there is little to no improvement within a few months of starting cyclic tVNS, the most interfering factor as a relapse of the intestinal bacterial or some other interfering supplement, or a homeopathic remedy, probiotics, recurrent herpes simplex, chronic dental infection or high dosages of vitamins or minerals.

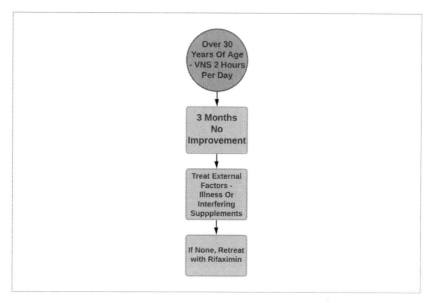

Adjustment of Therapy Patients Over 30 Years of Age

Increasing the tVNS above two hours per day will not solve these problems and should not be attempted. tVNS should never be programmed or conducted by yourself without the specific guidance of your physician. The vagus nerve is capable of being permanently damaged if stimulated improperly.

Caution: Because of the potential danger in the misuse of vagus nerve stimulation, vagus stimulation should not be attempted without the specific guidance of a physician experienced and knowledgeable with vagus nerve stimulation.

Time Course for VNS Therapy

At the time of publication of this book, the specific number of years of tVNS therapy required for children with autism or any form of developmental issue is unknown while data is collected on the children under my care who have been on tVNS long enough to determine if, or what kind, of relapse might occur if tVNS is discontinued after recovery.

In my view, the two primary effects of tVNS are to first restore neurological pruning, which helps the child develop and mature, and secondly to help repair damage to the autonomic nervous system and neural networks that occur from cumulative brain injury.

It is believed that the developmental pruning process during childhood is unidirectional meaning that once the child has have pruned off a branch of a neuron just like a branch of a tree, they can not replace it with a new one and increase the number of unorganized neurons again.

I do not think a child would regress from a developmental milestone standpoint if tVNS were discontinued (i.e., a child who has regained speech or socialization skills would not lose these skills once the brain is properly pruned). At the time of this writing, I am not aware of any of my patients developmentally regressing after tVNS has been discontinued.

My research using tVNS as part of The Nemechek Protocol® in adults for recovery autonomic dysfunction from cumulative brain injury demonstrates that after discontinuing tVNS, many adults will have a return of some of their autonomic symptoms (constipation, fidgetiness, headaches, poor focus) they experienced previously. Yet many also become less consistent with the other components of the protocol at the same time, so it is unknown if the symptoms return because of the absence of any single particular component or because of the combined deficiency of several.

This return of symptoms occurs slowly and is often apparent within four to eight weeks. In addition to a return of their symptoms, evidence of their prior autonomic damage as measured by autonomic spectral analysis will also return on repeat testing.

Therefore, once a child patient has reached developmental maturity and is behaving in a neurotypical fashion, I would consider discontinuation of tVNS while continuing fish oil, olive oil, and maintenance of intestinal bacteria balance with either inulin or rifaximin.

Either the recovery from cumulative brain injury (resolution of ADD, hyperactivity, anxiety, aggression, constipation, heartburn) will persist or they might notice a return of some of these symptoms within the eight weeks after discontinuation.

If the symptoms do not return, then the tVNS is no longer required. If a child seems to be relapsing, then re-initiation of tVNS is warranted.

If the child also has another non-developmental health condition (inflammatory bowel disease, epilepsy, or cerebral palsy) that also has improved because of the addition of tVNS, then I would not be in such a hurry to stop tVNS because these other conditions are often more than likely to return with discontinuation of tVNS.

PART IV

THE UPS AND DOWNS OF
RECOVERY

12

THE PROCESS OF RECOVERY

Parents often ask, "How fast does it take for the brain to recover?" The brain recovers as fast as hair grows. Every day your hair looks the same length until, after a few months, you suddenly realize that you need a haircut.

The process of reversal and recovery of the key features of autism and developmental disorders is a journey full of ups and downs. Gains in one particular aspect may be followed by the development of a new unusual behavior and it can be very frustrating for parents.

As I watch patients recover, I remind myself that various aspects of their nervous systems can be delayed by differing amounts. A child potentially could be delayed in socialization by only one year, motor function by two years, but speech by four years. This does not include the additional delay in forming the neural networks required for maturity.

Once recovery begins, a wide range of imbalances can present themselves and manifest as new abnormal behavior that might be misconstrued as a regression. I have even seen young adults in their 20's seeming go through their "terrible two's" as they recover.

The Awakening Period

As I mentioned in chapter 1, the first change I see during the first few weeks with my young patients is what I have described as "the awakening" period, an increased level of awareness and functioning due to the initial decline of the toxic effects of the propionic acid. The awakening can both improve and worsen certain behaviors. But from this point going forward, normal neuronal pruning begins the process of gradual neurological development and maturation and the child will begin improving month by month, year by year.

It helps to view a child with autism as a child who is under the effects of a sedative such as Valium (diazepam) or even alcohol. All their behaviors are blunted or subdued, they may seem calmer and sleep through the night, but they do not respond when spoken to, may seldom speak, and may not be aware of their surroundings.

In the case of autism, the sedative affecting the children is the elevated blood and tissue levels of propionic acid made by the overgrowth of bacteria within the child's small intestine which then leaks into the bloodstream. Reversing the bacterial overgrowth essentially reduces the sedating propionic acid from their body, and the child becomes more cognitively alert.

Children in the awakening period become aware of their surroundings. They are often more tolerant of being touched or held, are often more willing to approach someone and be physically closer to them. They may also be more active and communicate more, but may sometimes seem more anxious or sleep less.

The older the child, the less obvious the awakening period will be and children with only developmental issues and no diagnosis of autism will not have an awakening at all since they do not produce propionic acid.

After the first few weeks of the awakening period, recovery rates are highly variable due to the degree of developmental delay underlying each patient's toxic encephalopathy state. If the inflammatory cytokine process has been going on since birth, the child will be obviously experiencing more difficulties, unlike a child who is developing normally until their regressive event at eighteen months for instance.

Children starting the protocol in their teens will have a much greater degree of cumulative brain injury to overcome than a child starting the protocol at the age of five for instance.

If the inflammation is mild, the developmental delay often is relatively mild, and the children often regain function rather quickly. With very early and intense inflammation, there can be so much developmental delay or even developmental arrest that the child is diagnosed with global delay or mental retardation.

Despite this, I have children under my care who fit this description and are recovering as anticipated. While it will take longer for these more advanced cases, I do not believe their developmental challenges are insurmountable.

The True Extent of Brain Dysfunction

If the child also has underlying brain injuries from physical, emotional, or inflammatory traumas, parents may see more angry outbursts, hyperactivity, anxiety, and stimulation behavior after the awakening period.

This is because the sedating effect of propionic acid has suppressed these behaviors and as the propionic acid levels decline with the reversal of bacterial overgrowth, the behaviors become more apparent. Parents may observe a child who is the size of a fourteen-year old whose emotional capability is equivalent to a three-year old, or a child who can type but not speak.

The overriding point is that the change of behaviors after the awakening period is often not the worsening of underlying neurological problems, it is a glimpse of the true degree of underlying damage and developmental delay because the sedative effects of propionic acid that dampened their overall behavior is finally gone. The children are not worse, they are finally awake.

For some parents, this stage may be more challenging than others because the underlying behaviors are more disruptive to the household. After reducing bacterial overgrowth, new development and repair are dependent on consistently reducing inflammation with fish oil, COOC-certified California olive oil, decreasing the omega-6 vegetable oils from the diet, and incorporating vagus nerve stimulation when necessary.

With time these behaviors will begin improving because a child's brain has an enormous capacity to recover. One twenty-three-year old non-verbal ASD young adult patient I care for was finally able to start speaking in both Spanish and English after eight months, but only after going through a period of angry outbursts on the school bus, experiencing increased anxiety when she was sitting still, and after going through spells of having tantrums in the grocery store.

Once her propionic levels declined, she was in a place developmentally where she had tantrums lying on the floor crying like any other three-year-old in the grocery store when her parents would tell her to put an item back on the shelf. Her angry outbursts and anxiety on the school bus were from the lingering autonomic nervous system dysfunction that triggered her "fight or flight" feelings if she sat still for too long.

The Pace of Recovery

The important point to remember is that a child's brain has an enormous capacity to continue the path of development once the inflammation is consistently controlled. Neuronal and synaptic pruning will re-initiate, with some children able to catch-up about two to three months of development for every one calendar month. Most children will require more time than this and I unfortunately cannot predict the time frame for parents.

I am frequently asked what else might someone do to speed the healing. I tell parents to think of the brain repair process like someone wanting to speed up the recovery of their broken arm. A broken arm will not heal any faster by doing anything "extra." It is the same with brain recovery.

Bone tissue, like brain tissue, has its own naturally determined rate of recovery and there is no known way to improve upon the natural rate. I also tell parents not to compare their child's behavior today with yesterday, but instead compare them today to how they were one or two months ago, or when they first started the protocol.

Keeping a longer timeframe for the assessment of recovery is important because it prevents a parent from getting distracted by some of the common ups and downs in the recovery process.

Over Focusing and Misinterpreting

Some of the first changes to occur after starting the protocol might be in a child's skin condition or in the speed of the digestive tract. Usually if a child has eczema or psoriasis, the skin will noticeably improve. The Nemechek Protocol® will reverse bacterial overgrowth and this can lead to a resolution in diarrhea or sometimes a perceived worsening of constipation.

In patients with autism, the initial positive signs after rebalancing of the intestinal tract often is a reduction in anxiety (better sleep, less anxiety, less stimming), a greater awareness with their surroundings (improved eye-to-eye contact, recognizing the arrival of a familiar person) or are more awake or alert (less napping, wake up earlier, increased mental activity and engagement). These are signs that the propionic acid levels are dropping.

Some parents will over-focus on a smaller issue (constipation, bowel movement characteristics, giggling more, waking up earlier, holding hands over ears, moodiness, etc.) and interpret such an event as being bad or negative instead of a phase in healing. Parents want their children to talk but the lack of rapid speech improvement is also not an indication that balancing of the intestinal tract failed. Over-focusing in this manner may cause a parent to miss the bigger picture that this is just one step in the child's gradual improvement.

Behavior-Age Mismatch

Parents need to anticipate that their children's emotional maturity generally will not match their physical age during recovery. They may have an autistic child who is six, twelve, or twenty-four years old but behaves as if they are a two-year-old child.

They must do their best to be patient during this difficult time because in six months a child who behaved liked a two-year-old child may begin behaving as if they are three or four years old. In another six to twelve months, they may progress to the behavior of a five or six-year-old. This maturation process will continue on more or less over time.

Constipation, Stimming and Autonomic Dysfunction

The autonomic nervous system (ANS) is a large portion of the nervous system that controls and coordinates all organ function, emotional regulation, metabolism, hormonal production, and most of the immune system.

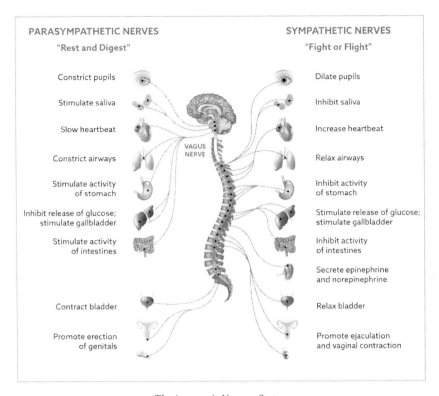

PARASYMPATHETIC NERVES
"Rest and Digest"

Constrict pupils
Stimulate saliva
Slow heartbeat
Constrict airways
Stimulate activity
of stomach
Inhibit release of glucose;
stimulate gallbladder
Stimulate activity
of intestines

Contract bladder

Promote erection
of genitals

VAGUS
NERVE

SYMPATHETIC NERVES
"Fight or Flight"

Dilate pupils
Inhibit saliva
Increase heartbeat
Relax airways
Inhibit activity
of stomach
Stimulate release of glucose;
stimulate gallbladder
Inhibit activity
of intestines
Secrete epinephrine
and norepinephrine
Relax bladder

Promote ejaculation
and vaginal contraction

The Autonomic Nervous System

In a child, the same inflammatory process that prevents the brain from properly developing will also prevent the brain from repairing damage to the autonomic nervous system from head banging, accidental falls, intense emotional traumas, or inflammatory trauma from surgery, allergy testing, or an adverse vaccine reaction.

The residual damage from prior injuries will add to the damage from new injuries in a process known as cumulative brain injury (CBI). Cumulative brain injuries will ultimately lead to enough autonomic nervous system damage that the child will experience symptoms. The same inflammation also impairs the development of neural networks that are required in order to develop into a mature eighteen-year-old.

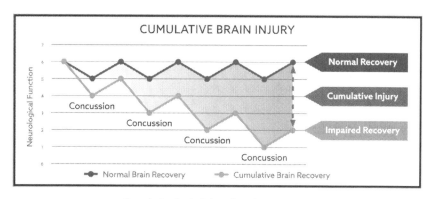

Cumulative Brain Injury from Brain Injuries

A very common problem after the reversal of bacterial overgrowth is the appearance of constipation in children. The brain controls the movement of the digestive tract, like a conveyor belt, through the autonomic nervous system.

From an autonomic viewpoint, constipation is the inability of the nervous system to push the contents of the stool forward on that conveyor belt and is a common symptom that develops after a physical brain injury. It is important to understand inulin or rifaximin do not "cause" constipation. It unmasks a pre-existing problem with the autonomic nervous system that is often the true cause of constipation.

Studies in adults find that 50-70% of adults will develop constipation within the first week after a mild-to-moderate concussion (i.e., head injury). The source of constipation is often the brain and nervous system, not the colon itself.

Understanding the mechanics that move the digestive tract helps parents understand the changes that they see in their child during the treatment of the bacterial overgrowth. Bacterial overgrowth may lead to either constipation, diarrhea (an increased rate of stool production), stool urgency, heartburn after particular foods, frequent bowel movements, or all the above.

If a child has an increased rate of stool production from bacterial overgrowth (i.e., diarrhea) while at the same time has inadequate forward stool propulsion from autonomic nervous system damage (i.e., constipation), they may seem to have a normal stool pattern. The liquid stool of diarrhea essentially treats the slow movement of stool in constipation.

Not understanding that this somewhat normal stool pattern may just be from two opposing imbalances that together present a "false" normal bowel pattern and can lead to improper decisions. Therefore, once the bacterial overgrowth is rebalanced and corrected with either inulin or rifaximin, the child's constipation suddenly seems to "be caused by" these therapies.

In fact, what happens is that the diarrhea (an underlying bacterial overgrowth problem) simply resolved thereby making the underlying constipation (an autonomic nervous system problem) more obvious. Eventually, the underlying constipation will slowly improve as the patient's autonomic nervous system recovers.

The Nemechek Protocol® steadily shifts the patient's microglia into repair mode, reducing brain inflammation, and stimulating brain stem cell production. When the microglia begin to function and the inflammation declines, the repair of the autonomic nervous system begins in earnest. It is the improvement of autonomic nervous system function that allows the digestive conveyor belt to move more naturally again.

Supplements and Prescription Medicine

I believe that a child with autism or developmental disorders should be under the primary supervision of a licensed physician who should always be consulted about any medicines or supplements recommended to the child by any other healthcare provider (physician, naturopath, DAN doctor, herbalist, etc.). No prescribed medicines or supplements should ever be reduced or stopped without permission and upon the direction of the prescribing physician.

I also believe that children are being over-treated with an enormous number of supplements for oxidative stress, mitochondrial defects, digestion, biofilm, folate problems, yeast overgrowth, parasites, and other metabolic disturbances.

Although many of those types of supplements may have improved something initially, they do not have a significant impact on the overall pattern of bacterial overgrowth, brain injury symptoms, and autonomic nervous system dysfunction that are such key features of autism and developmental delay. In my experience, many are capable of impeding or even reversing recovery. I have seen the removal of just one supplement finally bring about the healing process in the patient.

The Nemechek Protocol® does not use any of those types of products because none of them have any impact on either the reversal of bacterial overgrowth, microglial activation, or excessive levels of brain inflammation.

In my experience, the excessive use of supplements that are commonly prescribed to children with autism and developmental issues do not solve these target problems. If they did reverse these problems, the children would be experiencing significant recovery as is commonly reported after starting my protocol.

The reasons why many are ineffective is because many of these products are often only addressing the downstream effects of the much larger and overwhelming issue of metabolic inflammation.

Metabolic inflammation is the term used to describe the broad adverse effects that the chronic elevation of pro-inflammatory cytokines has on cellular function. Metabolic inflammation must be persistently lowered for cells to begin functioning more normally.

I often speak of metabolic inflammation as if it is water flooding a valley because the dam upstream is broken and it no longer holds back the water. When the dam breaks the homes and fields downstream of the dam become flooded from the excessive flow of water.

The water in my example is meant to represent the massive release of pro-inflammatory cytokines associated with bacterial overgrowth, the deficiency of the dietary omega-3 fatty acids, the excessive dietary intake of omega-6 fatty acid-rich oils and foods, and often damage to the inflammation-controlling vagus nerve.

Certain efforts, such as placing sandbags around a home or pumping water out of a basement, may provide some benefit to the flooded area but they do not address the primary problem which is the broken dam. Sandbags and basement pumps are like many of the supplements used to address mitochondrial dysfunction or the depletion of antioxidants. The real problem remains. The dam needs to be repaired and once that occurs, the sandbags and basement pumps are no longer required.

Once there is a reduction of metabolic inflammation with The Nemechek Protocol® in my patients, I see the need for supplements addressing mitochondrial dysfunction and antioxidant depletion disappear.

> *Regarding all prescription medications or prescription supplements (e.g. iron, Vitamin D3, injectable Vitamin B12, or leucovorin), parents should never under any circumstance reduce or stop those without first consulting their child's managing physician.*

Understanding Bacterial Terminology

Our understanding of the diversity of microbes living within the human intestinal tract is rapidly expanding, and a few phrases (dysbiosis, low biodiversity, SIBO, and bacterial overgrowth) may seem similar but are all slightly different from each other.

Dysbiosis is a general term referring to any change in the blend of living microbes within the intestinal tract. It does not specifically apply to only bacteria and it may refer to viruses, protozoan, or archaebacteria.

In addition to an imbalance of one type or species of a micro-organism to another, dysbiosis may also refer to the absence of certain species thought to normally inhabit the human intestinal tract. The extinction or loss of species is referred to as low biodiversity.

SIBO (small intestinal bacterial overgrowth) implies the patient has an overgrowth of bacteria within the small intestine. These typically are common bacteria that normally live down in the colon (the lower intestinal tract); they are just living up in the wrong place.

The "gold standard" test for determining bacterial overgrowth is a procedure that requires a long endoscope to be passed into the small intestine in order to sample bacteria within the jejunum portion of the small intestine. Then the sample needs to undergo quantitative culturing, DNA identification, and metabolic activation testing of the species in the sample.

I do not recommend that any of my patients undergo the gold standard test as it is expensive, impractical, is not available outside of a research study, and is unnecessary in order to achieve improvement using The Nemechek Protocol®.

Some people undergo a "SIBO breath test" looking for a SIBO diagnosis but the breath test is prone to many sources of error. Within my practice, I stopped using SIBO breath testing on my patients to determine overgrowth because unacceptably high false positive and false negative results made it clinically useless.

Also, we know that all children with autism must have bacterial overgrowth in order to produce propionic acid or trigger inflammatory primed microglia, so why perform a test when we already know the answer. In order to reverse the damaging effect of autism, bacterial balance must be restored, or the children simply fail to improve.

The Misconception of Feeding "Bad" Bacteria and Yeast with Inulin

It is difficult to imagine the hundreds of thousands of bacteria within our digestive tract that are causing our brains and bodies so much trouble. Common questions from parents of my patients are whether inulin feeds "bad bacteria" and yeast.

Inulin is a safe prebiotic fiber that produces enough bacterial rebalancing, propionic acid reduction, and inflammation reduction to allow a child to become more alert and restart the process of neuronal pruning and development.

Inulin is present in large amounts in garlic and onions and these foods have been historically safe to feed children over many millennia. Combining inulin with fish oil and olive oil is nothing more than the same ingredients a child might have eaten in ancient Rome.

I generally recommend starting with inulin in patients who are children because it is often effective, safe, inexpensive, and does not require a prescription to obtain. Inulin is widely available from several manufacturers. Inulin is also appealing as a natural fiber that many parents prefer who are understandably fearful of using any more antibiotics.

If a child's parents are worried about using inulin because of the fear of feeding "bad bacteria," I recommend they use rifaximin to eliminate the bacterial overgrowth. This moves them beyond the issue of "good" and "bad" bacteria that seem to be holding some people back from starting my regimen. Rifaximin seems to work as well as inulin in children.

The misrepresentations that increased stimming, less sleeping, or increased anxiety is from inulin feeding "bad" bacteria have been concerns of parents in the past. I agree that symptoms may worsen by changes in the diet, but I do not believe that this is the case with inulin. I have not seen any indication that inulin increases bacterial overgrowth in any of my patients.

I believe there are several reasons for this. **The first reason** is that inulin's main effect is within the lumen of the small intestine where bacteria digest inulin through a process referred to as fermentation. The primary effect of fermentation is the production of a healthy short-chain fatty acid known as butyric acid. Only small amounts of inulin pass through to the colon and if it does it is digested to form a harmless gas.

The second reason why I do not believe inulin feeds bad bacteria or yeast is that a significant increase in pathogenic bacteria, or overgrowth of bacteria, would almost certainly cause an increase in diarrhea, stool frequency, abdominal cramping, reflux, and eczema. I do not see those reactions in my patients, in fact, I see a general reversal of those symptoms with the use of inulin.

If the intestinal (not neurological or behavioral) symptoms were to worsen on inulin, I would assess whether the worsening symptoms are from some other underlying condition such as a viral infection or possibly inflammatory bowel disease. If uncertain, I generally will suggest discontinuing the inulin to be 100% certain.

If the diarrhea does not stop, then I would recommend consultation with a pediatric gastroenterologist to look for another cause such as inflammatory bowel disease. If the diarrhea stops and recurs with discontinuation and resumption of inulin, I will then prescribe rifaximin and discontinue the inulin altogether.

Remember, the development of constipation with the use of inulin is a sign of underlying autonomic nervous system dysfunction from developmental and cumulative brain injury that typically reverses after a few months of diligent fish oil, EVOO, and a reduction in dietary omega-6 oils.

The third reason why I do not believe that inulin feeds bad bacteria or yeast is that propionic acid has a sedating effect on children, almost as if the children had been taking Valium or Xanax. Therefore, once inulin reverses the bacterial overgrowth and the propionic acid levels decline, I see the children come out of their stupor.

Their different behavior during or after the awakening period is the result of their pre-existing and underlying developmental abnormalities, cumulative brain injuries, and autonomic dysfunction. I do not believe their behavior is from any toxic effect of inulin, as I have seen these behaviors improve or stop over time while the patient is on their continued inulin.

A fourth reason why I do not believe that inulin feeds bad bacteria or yeast is that the detection of pathogenic bacteria such as Klebsiella in the stool (a sample of bacteria within the colon, not the small intestine) by no means suggests that these bacteria are present within the small intestine where inulin has its main effect.

The detection of pathogenic bacteria such as *Klebsiella pneumoniae* or *Clostridium difficle* is commonly found in asymptomatic patients and is essentially harmless. Their growth is kept in check by a healthy balance of other bacteria which is further bolstered with inulin. In addition, some parents are worried about the overgrowth of candida.

I agree that candida and other yeasts (also known as fungi) inhabit the intestinal tract, but many in-depth studies demonstrate that yeast (fungal) overgrowth does not occur in autism nor does it cause "leaky gut." The symptoms that have been misattributed to candida or yeast are instead the consequence of bacterial overgrowth.

Finally, while the observations of clinical improvement after the reduction of sugars and carbohydrates (think GF/CF, FODMAPS, GAPS) are true, these are also misattributed to yeast. The clinical improvement is instead due to a "starving effect" from the reduction in carbohydrates while on these diets. Fewer dietary sugars and carbohydrates leads to diminished growth of bacteria which in turn leads to diminished production of propionic acids and ultimately the clinical improvement in the children.

Intestinal Symptoms and Stool Testing

When children are experiencing occasional intestinal issues, I always consider whether some other common mechanism is causing their intestinal symptoms.

Things to consider include viral infections, injury to the autonomic nervous system, reaction to other medications or supplements, or tainted food. Adverse reactions to these events should resolve within one to two weeks without necessitating changes in dosage or the discontinuation of inulin.

Occasionally, patients have chronic diarrhea, loose stools, or an oily film in the stool. These things generally occur for two reasons. The first is that their intestinal tract is injured or stressed from the bacterial overgrowth. Their intestinal tract will begin to repair itself within two to three weeks after starting inulin or treatment with a course of rifaximin. Because of the rapid healing, patients do not need any special "gut-healing" supplements or special diets.

The second reason is that their intestines may not be accustomed to absorbing the volume of oil used on The Nemechek Protocol®. The intestinal tract alters its ability to absorb oils depending on the amount of oil in the person's diet.

To improve oil absorption in my patients, I first decrease their amounts of fish oil and EVOO to a lower dose that allows their stools to normalize somewhat. Then, I have them slowly increase their dose of fish oil, followed by olive oil a little every week until reaching the full dose in about three to four weeks.

Although testing the stool for bacteria and yeast is commonly performed by other practitioners, I urge a word of caution to my patients at their interpretation. The first issue is that approximately 90% of the bacterial species that live within the intestine are not able to be grown by common laboratory techniques.

Culture results from a stool specimen will only potentially grow 10% of all the species present. Drawing a conclusion about the balanced health of the intestinal bacterial blend from only 10% of the population is bound to be inaccurate. Accurate identification of bacteria species can only be done by quantitative DNA sequencing techniques.

The second issue is that a stool sample coming from the last part of the colon contains a vastly different blend of bacteria and cannot be compared to a sample aspirated from the small intestine. The negative health effects from bacterial overgrowth are due to excessive bacteria growing in the small intestine, not the colon.

Analysis for bacterial overgrowth of the small intestine (SIBO) requires a sample of fluid from within the small intestine and this sample can only be obtained by an endoscopy (EGD; esophagogastroduodenoscopy) and is generally only performed for research purposes. Because of the complexity, cost and risk to the patient, I do not recommend obtaining samples by endoscopy.

On rare occasions, a simple stool testing might detect parasitic organisms called protozoans (like Giardia) or helminths (worms). Detection of one of these organisms might require treatment depending on the organism found, the nature of the patient's symptoms, and the potential adverse effects of the treatment. Infection with these types of organisms tend to occur when consuming contaminated water or foods or by walking barefoot in areas that are contaminated.

The Risk of Running Unnecessary Tests

By the time most people come to my office for a consultation, many have been misled, over-charged, and even harmed physically and emotionally by excessive and unnecessary laboratory tests (enzymes, food intolerance, infectious disease antibody levels, metabolic panels, genetic panels) or physical testing (CT/MRI scans, EEG, etc.).

The modern era of medicine has seen an excessive dependence on the ordering of a wide variety of tests to help determine the cause of the patient's symptoms. The interactions with providers can easily become nothing more than a timely and expensive guessing game. The traditional and most effective method of diagnostics in medicine is a thorough history and examination to determine the most probable cause of a person's symptoms.

As an internal medicine doctor, I was taught that a clinician should not order any testing until they have determined the one or two conditions that are most likely responsible for the patient's symptoms. Any tests that are run should be specific to either rule in or rule out these conditions. A common example I see is when a clinician orders several different antibody panels looking for a variety of different organisms, all of which would cause vastly different symptoms. When I see this in a patient's medical records, I know the other doctor is lost diagnostically.

Tests ordered should be based on the patient's particular symptoms. If the patient is not exhibiting symptoms suggestive of EBV or Babesiosis, these antibody levels should never be ordered. An unnecessary test can return a false positive result and now the entire clinical treatment strategy is moving down the wrong path.

Broad panels of tests for random things that do not change the patient's course of care should always be avoided. The question I ask myself when ordering tests is whether the test result will change the treatment strategy that I have planned for the patient.

Procedures such as colonoscopies, MRI scans, or EEG should only be ordered if the results will alter the course of treatment. These tests should never be performed simply to "take a look" because they all have the potential to harm the child physically and emotionally.

Restricting Foods in the Diet

I do not restrict any foods in the diet when I treat my patients with The Nemechek Protocol® other than foods known to cause severe allergic reactions (peanuts, walnuts, etc.) or obvious intolerance (milk causing diarrhea, etc.) in the patient.

The benefits that occur in autistic patients after starting any diet that restricts carbohydrates (GAPS, FODMAPS, gluten, casein, etc.) are often from the relative, non-specific decrease in the overall bacterial load within the intestinal tract. The bulk of intestinal bacteria thrive on carbohydrates and a decrease in bacterial counts occurs with a decrease in dietary carbohydrates.

If a child has been on a restrictive diet of some sort prior to starting The Nemechek Protocol®, I recommend reintroducing the restricted foods a few weeks after starting the inulin or after completing the course of rifaximin.

Obvious exceptions to this are foods such as peanuts that may have caused a severe allergic reaction previously in the child. These should never be re-introduced. If there are any questions about the severity of past food reactions, I recommend the parent discuss this with their primary care physician.

Unfortunately, many children have developed a limited pattern of food preferences (the so-called picky eaters). While this can be frustrating and worrisome for parents, it resolves on its own over time.

I recommend against adding vitamins to "make sure they get everything they need." The importance of a wide variety of foods is less critical than most people think and the high rate of fraud in the supplement industry provides the potential for harm. This is one of the major reasons I advise against supplementing with vitamins.

Some studies suggest the symptoms of gluten intolerance seems to occur because of an abnormal inflammatory reaction against gluten. This inflammatory reaction may be the result of parasympathetic weakness of the autonomic nervous system and not directly related to bacterial translocation (leaky gut).

As the child starts recovering neurologically, the autonomic nervous system begins to recover, and gluten intolerance often slowly resolves without needing to remain on a gluten-free diet.

Physical, Occupational and Speech Therapies

I agree with continuing any form of occupational or physical therapy while a patient is on The Nemechek Protocol® but, as the child improves, I think many of these therapies become unnecessary and can trigger negative behaviors in the children.

Humans are a species that evolved to walk, talk, and socialize and our ability to prune our brain is predetermined by nature no differently than a bird's brain develops and understands how to build a nest.

My experience has taught me that once the child is showing overall signs of neurological recovery on The Nemechek Protocol® and they have overcome their primary obstacle with therapy, the therapy should be stopped and the child given the opportunity to recover on their own. Common social interactions with parents, siblings and others is ample stimulation to allow for continued normal development.

During the pandemic when schools were closed and children were no longer receiving the variety of therapies, many children under my care experienced continued gains and sometime gains much greater that seen when actively getting therapy.

Monitoring Propionic Acid Levels

Although there are tests available that can measure propionic acid levels in the bloodstream and urine, there are no set standards we can use to determine if a level is too high or low in a manner similar to our interpretation of blood sugar (glucose) levels. Therefore, I do not order any testing for propionic acid for my patients.

Furthermore, there are a variety of metabolic variants of propionic acid (3HHA, 3HPA, HPHPA) and no one really knows whether they should be used as a marker for autism.

There is no reason to test for propionic acid to guide therapy. We already know that the non-autistic child will not have propionic acid effects, while the autistic child will. My treatment for both children is the same, with or without the presence of propionic acid.

In addition, I suspect in ten years or more we will have discovered that chemicals other than propionic acid can potentially be released by the overgrowth of bacteria and that these can also lead to behavioral changes. Remember, a major aspect of The Nemechek Protocol® is to reverse the bacterial overgrowth in the small intestine, and this would predictable eliminate the production of any chemical from the overgrowing bacteria.

Successful rebalancing of the intestinal bacteria will result in the reduction of both inflammatory stress as well as the reduction in the abnormal production of chemicals whether it is propionic acid or something else.

If a child under my care has any features resembling autism, any spectral disorder, ADD/ ADHD, a mood disorder, or any form of developmental delay I will start them on The Nemechek Protocol® because with any of these diagnoses the patient has a good chance of improvement or recovery regardless of a propionic-related test result.

My protocol is focused on restoring neurological function through the reduction of inflammation within the nervous system. All of these conditions will similarly improve because they all occur as a result of the lack of proper neuronal pruning, repair and rejuvenation mechanisms.

The Genetic Wildcard in Recovery

Broadly speaking autism was previously believed to be a predominantly genetic disorder. This belief is eroding away as more and more evidence highlights the importance of bacterial overgrowth as a triggering phenomenon for most autism and developmental delay.

Since a child's intestinal bacteria blend comes from his or her mother, it is easy to understand how researchers of the past may have noted a tendency for autism to occur more in one family more than another. We are now beginning to understand it is not the passage of a parent's genetic material that is driving autism, it is often the passage of a damaged gut microbiome from mother to child.

In spite of this, many children with autism will often undergo genetic testing to help focus the diagnosis of their developmental disorder. The problem with this random genetic testing is twofold.

First, the specter of a "genetic disorder" implies it is irreversible and leaves many parents feeling that recovery is impossible. In fact, many parents are being counseled that because of these genetic test results, there is little hope for their child to improve.

Secondly, demonstrating there is a genetic abnormality does not mean the abnormality is a *cause* of autism. Some genetic abnormalities in autistic children can be found in a certain percentage of all children with autism. This still does not mean that the identified genes "cause" autism.

There is a very real possibility that some of these genes with a high association with autism may simply trigger bacterial overgrowth or lead to a predilection of overgrowth with a propionic acid producing bacterium. I believe this is more common than not and explains why so many children improve on my protocol in spite of their genetic abnormality.

Another fact is that finding a gene for any particular medical condition does not mean the gene is necessarily active. A common example is that many people with brown eyes may be carrying a gene for blue eyes. They have the gene for blue eyes, but it has not been activated. I have seen a wide variety of children recovering with The Nemechek Protocol® despite tests demonstrating the presence of abnormal genes or genetic deletions.

While the anatomic issues (small cranium, musculoskeletal issues with arms or legs, etc.) associated with some of these genetic abnormalities do not improve, I have seen the majority of these children experience significant neurological gains with The Nemechek Protocol®.

The Other Children in the Family

In reviewing a patient's medical history, many provide a family history suggesting symptoms of intestinal dysbiosis beginning a few generations prior to the child with autism.

The intestinal bacteria of each maternal generation is damaged by antibiotics, preservatives, pesticides, microplastics, and then passed on to the next generation. These cycles of accumulated intestinal bacterial damage continue with each generation.

This results in a progressive decline in biodiversity and as the biodiversity declines, the body's ability to maintain the separation of bacteria between the small intestine ("birds") and colon ("fish") weakens further. It is important to remember that the low biodiversity contributes to the unstable intestinal bacteria balance that if lost, triggers the cascade resulting in autism, many developmental disorders as well as cumulative brain injury.

Therefore, since the child who has autism or developmental issues received their low biodiversity blend from their mother, all non-adopted siblings will have a somewhat similar risk of developing bacterial overgrowth as well. I believe all children from the same family may benefit from my protocol.

The protocol is extremely safe and I believe has a good chance of preventing the other children in the family (who have similar low biodiversity) from developing autism, developmental delay or developing ADD, headaches, or depression later on in childhood.

13

MANAGING ANXIETY TANTRUMS, OCD AND AGGRESSION

I n my pursuit to help reverse patients' health problems, I try to identify the underlying mechanisms driving these problems rather than prescribing medications that often just mask the problems. Masking or controlling symptoms with medications is not necessarily improper nor should it be considered "bad" medicine; often it is the best we can do with the scientific knowledge at hand.

However, many chronic conditions are the result of excessive inflammation, and unbalanced intestinal bacteria is often a contributing source of the inflammation. Typical medications used to treat these conditions only treat the downstream effects from inflammatory damage but not the underlying source of inflammation.

A big difference between treating children (especially kids with a communication disability) and adults is that children often do not talk about symptoms they are experiencing or they might not be able to communicate their symptoms in the same manner that most adults can.

For example, a child might have a simple runny nose and an occasional cough for a few weeks but because there is no high fever their symptoms are often interpreted as allergies or a mild virus and no further evaluation is entertained.

An adult may have the same symptoms, but they can also volunteer that they have a headache, muscle aches, occasional chills, and a sore throat. The adult is then diagnosed as having a sinus infection and might be offered antibiotics or a nasal steroid spray. The child might have had the same additional symptoms but was simply did not provide these added pieces of clinical information that changed the entire treatment approach.

The same problem occurs when treating, diagnosing, and managing conditions like anxiety, tantrums (emotional fits), OCD-like behaviors, and overly aggressive reactions. Because we are unable to question the child about what they feel, it is often impossible to be sure what they are feeling (e.g., anxiety versus fear, frustration versus anger).

Because the clinical history is rather limited, I approach these problems from a mechanical-injury perspective. In other words, what neurological pathways may be broken to result in these behaviors? Anxiety and aggression can be very appropriate or inappropriate depending on whether truly threatening circumstances are present (e.g., being chased by a tiger) or not (e.g., sitting still for an extended period during school or a car ride). Appropriate reactions are often readily apparent and generally not of concern. Inappropriate reactions tend to be unpredictable and frustrating to the parents.

There are a variety of situations and physical conditions that can trigger the release of the "fight or flight" hormone noradrenaline (also known as norepinephrine). It is the release of this hormone that causes adults and children to feel anxious, aggressive, or fearful and causes them to want to flee from the triggering situation.

Rebalancing intestinal bacteria with inulin or rifaximin can sometimes result in a significant decline in anxiety and aggression. If the symptoms are persistent after rebalancing intestinal bacteria, the excessive emotional responses are most commonly due to unrepaired damage to the autonomic nervous system (cumulative brain injury).

Excessive emotional reactions can occur after rather severe injury to the limbic system of the central nervous system. In blast-induced neurotrauma experienced by soldiers, limbic system injuries are thought to be due to the combination of the concussion of the blast and the twisting of the head from the blast. Luckly, injury to the limbic system is otherwise very uncommon in routine concussions.

Some medications can trigger the release of fight-or-flight hormones if the medications lower blood pressure and oxygen delivery to the brain. Medications most capable of this include blood pressure-lowering medications used to try to control anxiety (clonidine, guanfacine, propranolol) as well as some psychotropic medications (risperidone).

The focus of this chapter is on the behaviors in children labeled as anxiety, panic attacks, OCD, or aggression that result from autonomic dysfunction.

A Mechanical View of Anxiety

As discussed elsewhere in the book, bacterial overgrowth in the small intestine results in three discreet pathological processes; the release of abnormal amounts of propionic acid, the release of pro-inflammatory cytokines and activation of an abnormal population of cells in the brain known as primed microglia.

While the release of propionic acid is responsible for a portion of features that are unique to autism (loss of eye contact and awareness), the pro-inflammatory cytokines and primed microglia both directly impair the brain's natural ability to prune and repair the brain.

Remember, cumulative brain injury (CBI) is the inability to fully repair the brain after mild to severe brain injuries leading to residual damage from a recent injury to be added to residual damage from past injuries. Although any portion of the brain can become damaged after a head trauma, damage to the autonomic nervous system often results in noticeable symptoms.

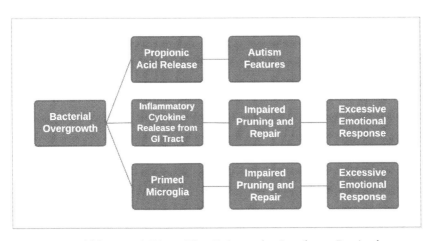

Bacterial Overgrowth Triggers Three Pathways that Contribute to Emotional Problems

The autonomic nervous system (ANS) controls all aspects of the body's involuntary physiological functioning. It controls the immune system, regulates hormone production, controls metabolism, the motility of the intestinal tract, blood pressure, heart rate as well as the proper intensity of emotional responses.

Furthermore, the autonomic nervous system can be injured through a variety of traumas other than just a physical injury. There is growing evidence that the brain can also sustain cellular damage after significant emotional traumas, or after the release of inflammatory cytokines from surgeries, fractures, vaccines, and even after a stroke within the brain. Any of these traumas have the potential to increase damage to the autonomic nervous system.

Mechanisms of Injury to the Nervous System

- **Physical Injury:** concussion or sub-concussive events

- **Inflammatory Injury:** surgery, vaccinations, fractures

- **Emotional Trauma:** moving to a new home, change in trusted therapist, bullying

The most common symptoms arising from brain injury result from the autonomic nervous system not being able to regulate blood pressure within the brain correctly and resulting in suboptimal pressure and oxygen delivery to the brain. The technical term for this is cerebral hypoperfusion.

The low brain pressure and inadequate release of oxygen commonly result in symptoms like headaches (migraine, cluster, or tension), chronic and unexplained fatigue, difficulty with concentration and focus (often diagnosed as ADD or ADHD), hyperactivity, insomnia, and increased thirst and/or hunger with particular cravings for salty or sweet foods.

Most importantly, low brain blood pressure can result in the periodic release of the fight or flight hormone noradrenaline. Noradrenaline is released from nerves of the sympathetic branch of the autonomic nervous system, not from the adrenal gland as its name might suggest.

As the phrase "fight or flight" suggests, noradrenaline can cause aggressive, anxious, and frightened behaviors that sometimes manifest as the need to escape or flee. This need to escape is often referred to as elopement in children. There is growing scientific evidence that children with autism, developmental disorders, and attention-learning deficits suffer from autonomic dysfunction and low brain blood pressure.

Anxious, Hungry, Hyperactive, and Aggressive Responses

The ANS has evolved in all animals including humans to help keep them alive in the wild. Primitive apes and stone-age humans had no modern concept of how much they needed to eat or drink, but they survived because the ANS would make them feel hungry or thirsty.

The ANS tells us to sleep and when to wake. The ANS scans the environment for signs of danger and constantly gives feedback about safety or danger. These signals are often referred to as our "sixth sense" or our "inner voice" when a situation strikes us in an uncomfortable manner.

If the ANS is injured, the loss of proper blood pressure and oxygen delivery to the brain is an urgent issue because the brain only has one second of reserve oxygen and is worried about passing out and dying from lack of oxygen. The urgency and physical reaction to the suboptimal oxygen supply can sometimes be as intense as one might feel if they were drowning. In order to survive, the brain will seek out ways to improve blood pressure and oxygen delivery.

The brain learns that liquids or foods containing salt or sugar will boost blood pressure to the head and help improve oxygen delivery to the neurons. This is what drives the incessant need in some children to eat or drink and if they do not get enough, they begin to act irritable and angry. Some parents jokingly refer to this combination of hungry and angry as "hangry."

Likewise, movement of the leg muscles will increase blood pressure and oxygen delivery to the brain. We have all witnessed an individual in a cafe or at a desk at work whose feet or legs are tapping or bouncing incessantly. In children with autism, the low blood pressure problem is responsible for their hyperactivity and toe-walking behaviors which through contraction of muscles, pushes blood upward into the brain.

The contraction of the leg muscles while moving or standing up on their tippy toes also helps squeeze blood flow upward towards the brain, improves oxygen delivery to neurons, and helps to dampen their uncontrollable fight or flight impulses.

The movement of the muscles is subconsciously driven by the brain to prevent itself from passing out and possibly dying. Some children will improve blood flow to their brain by lying flat or even hanging their heads upside down off the edge of a sofa or a bed.

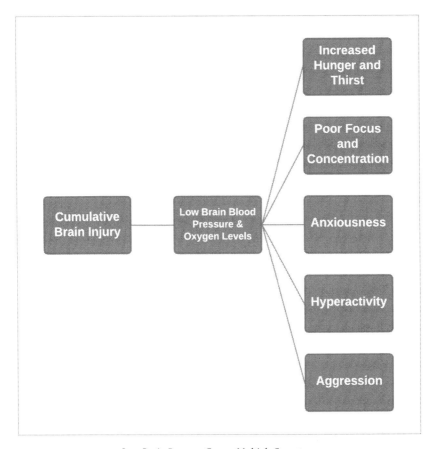

Low Brain Pressure Causes Multiple Symptoms

If a neurotypical seventh-grade boy sustains injuries that result in low brain blood pressure, he may act a little restless or fidgety in class and might be seen tapping his feet at times. If the brain pressure is low enough, it might affect his focus and concentration and he will be diagnosed with attention deficit disorder (ADD).

He may snack on some salty or sweet foods he has in his backpack. Although he's feeling restless, he doesn't get out of his chair. At his age and maturity level, he has enough impulse control to remain seated because he knows he will be in trouble with his teacher if he were to get up and wander about.

If that boy were in first grade instead of seventh grade, he would not be as able to control his impulses because of his immaturity. He would hop out of his chair whenever his brain needs to move his muscles to drive blood pressure and oxygen delivery. He is labeled as having hyperactivity unless he is also having trouble staying focused and paying attention then he will be labeled as having attention deficit and hyperactivity disorder.

An elementary-aged child once told me that when they sat in their chair too long their vision began to fade and would temporarily go completely black. What they are describing is the slow decline in oxygen delivery to the brain as their blood pressure slowly declines in their brain while sitting still.

The child understandably became anxious or frightened and would get up from their chair and move around the classroom to prevent this from recurring. To those observing the child, it seems as if they are misbehaving and not following instructions. But from the child's perspective, they are simply obeying the brain's command to use body movement to improve blood and oxygen delivery to the brain.

The impulse to move muscles is driven by the release of the fight or flight hormones. As their name implies, the primitive impulse the child experiences from the fight or flight hormones is extremely powerful and in addition to making the child restless and hyperactive, can cause them to also feel unusually anxious, fearful, angry, and aggressive.

Recognizing Low Blood Pressure Issues in Children with Autism or Developmental Disorders

The hyperactivity and anxiousness, anger, or aggression that I have just described is the same reason why young children with autism or developmental disorders have difficulty sitting still or focusing. It is often why some will suddenly pull hair, scratch, or bite when frustrated.

The same process that triggers autism and developmental issues is also responsible for the inadequate repair of brain trauma, cumulative brain injury, and the resulting low brain blood pressure. These children are often unable to sit still because their brain is fearful that they may die of lack of oxygen if they do.

They walk, toe walk, run, climb, and bounce to generate blood pressure in their brains. Some of the arm flapping might also be able to generate blood pressure to the head via the large upper arm blood vessels. Some of the children are constantly hungry or thirsty which will defy willpower or even the instruction of the parents to stop eating or drinking.

In my experience, the low blood pressure phenomenon is extremely common, and I will see it occur almost daily among families visiting me in my office. During a one-hour consultation, the child has had little to eat or drink and is somewhat restrained in their movement because of the size of my office.

Often, the child's anxious, disruptive, and aggressive behavior starts to escalate the longer the visit goes on. I often ask the parents to feed them something salty or sweet if available and encourage the child to drink about 2-4 oz. of water within five minutes. These simple steps increase blood pressure and oxygen delivery to the brain and relieve the fear of drowning that the brain was beginning to experience.

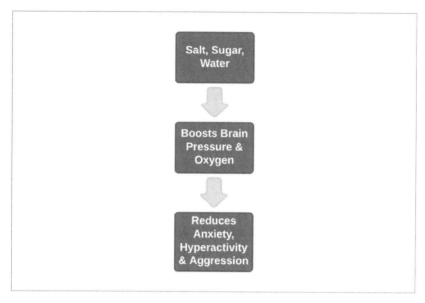

Salt, Sugar and Water Can Reduce Anxiety

There are other extenuating circumstances that can temporarily worsen a child's underlying brain blood pressure problems: lack of sleep, mild sinus or gastrointestinal infections, fever, emotionally stressful situations, and pain (dental or abdominal) are all able to temporarily worsen a child's blood pressure issues and trigger the symptoms I have described.

Sometimes Exercise, Salt, Sugar, and Water are Not Enough

Through practical experience, most parents learn that exercise, food, or liquids will help make their children better able to focus and less irritable or anxious. But sometimes the low brain blood pressure issues are to such an extent that these simple steps have little to no effect on helping calm their child. In certain circumstances, prescription medications can be used to control the anxiety, hyperactivity, or aggressive behaviors.

What and when to be used is best decided by the patient's managing physician. My discussion of these medications is intended as a guide for physicians and parents to understand the medications commonly used and this is not a particular recommendations for any of my patients on the protocol.

Behavior Control Medications Used in Autism and Developmental Disorders

- Benzodiazepine
- Antihistamines
- Serotonin Reuptake Inhibitors
- Alpha-2-Adrenergic-Agonist
- Anti-Psychotic Agents
- Blood Pressure Boosting Drugs

Typically, these medicines are chosen to suppress the anxious behavior irrespective of the cause of the anxiety. Anxiety can be suppressed using a class of medications known as serotonin reuptake inhibitors, such as fluoxetine (Prozac®) or sertraline (Zoloft®). Hydroxyzine (Antivert®) is an antihistamine prescribed to help with mild anxiety.

Also, more potent benzodiazepine medications, such as alprazolam (Xanax®), might be used for emergencies involving severe anxiety and aggression. These medicines can be highly effective but are to be used with caution because of the potential for addiction.

Some children are placed on alpha-2-adrenergic-agonist medications that traditionally have been used to lower anxiety for common daytime situations such as generalized anxiety and stage fright. Common examples include propranolol (Inderal®), guanfacine (Tenex®, Intuniv®), and clonidine (Catapres®).

Drugs that Reduce both Anxiety and Lower Blood Pressure

- Propranolol (Inderal®)
- Guanfacine (Tenex®, Intuniv®)
- Clonidine (Catapres®)

Ironically, these medicines were originally developed to lower blood pressure by blocking the effects of noradrenalin (norepinephrine). These medications are used with the intent of lowering anxiety in children by blocking the effects of noradrenaline but in doing so these medications can sometimes worsen anxiety and aggression by lowering the blood pressure in the brain even further. This may have the unintended effect of trapping the child in an emotional roller-coaster of fluctuating anxiety and aggression.

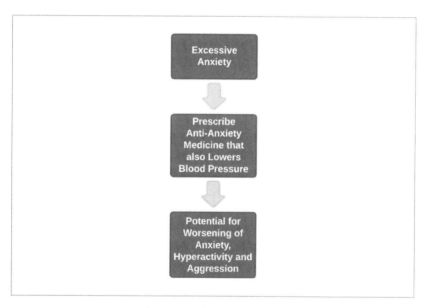

Potential Worsening of Anxiety with Medications

When there is more intense anxiety involving aggressive behavior, potent anti-psychotic medications are sometimes used. These medications work through uncertain mechanisms and are employed to simply control behaviors. These drugs can also cause severe side effects such as tardive dyskinesia, psychosis, and even suicide. I believe they should be prescribed only by physicians as a last resort. Some common examples are aripiprazole (Abilify®), quetiapine fumarate (Seroquel®), haloperidol (Haldol®), and risperidone (Risperidol®).

Children who respond to The Nemechek Protocol® should be closely monitored by their physicians so these medications may be properly adjusted and potentially tapered off as their autonomic nervous system recovers.

Boosting Blood Pressure to Reduce Anxiety and Aggression

Contrary to traditional anti-anxiety medications, I have found the use of medication to increase brain blood pressure to be very effective in reducing anxiety and aggression in many children.

Drugs that boost blood pressure have been known to help calm anxious, hyperactive children. The medicines used to boost blood pressure work by either stimulating the sympathetic branch of the autonomic nervous system (sympathomimetics) or by increasing the retention of saltwater in the body (fludrocortisone).

Several medicines (Ritalin®, Adderall®, and Concerta®) commonly used for attention deficit disorder (ADD) or attention deficit hyperactivity disorder (ADHD) improve the child's behavior by boosting blood pressure into the brain as well as directly stimulating the brain (similar to caffeine).

Drugs that Boost Blood Pressure and Stimulate the Brain
- Amphetamine/dextroamphetamine (Adderall®)
- Lisdexamfetamine dimesylate (Vyvanse®)
- Atomoxetine hydrochloride (Strattera®)
- Methylphenidate (Quillivant XR®)
- Methylphenidate (Focalin XR®)
- Methylphenidate (Concerta®)
- Methylphenidate (Ritalin®)
- Amphetamine (Dexedrine®)
- Amphetamine (Evekeo®)
- Droxidopa (Northera®)

Some children do not tolerate these drugs but there are other medications that boost blood pressure to the brain. Because they do not penetrate the central nervous system, they do not overstimulate children with autism or developmental disorders. My preference is to use a limited course of midodrine (Proamantine®) with my patients suffering from symptoms associated with low brain blood pressure.

Drugs that Only Boost Blood Pressure
- Midodrine (Proamantine®)
- Fludrocortisone (Florinef®)

Midodrine was approved in the U.S. for the treatment of low blood pressure (orthostatic hypotension) resulting from autonomic dysfunction in adults in 1996. The drug stimulates sympathetic receptors in the body and results in a boost of blood pressure upwards into the brain.

Adult patients with low blood pressure with autonomic dysfunction often feel anxious, have difficulty focusing or concentrating, have increased levels of hunger and thirst, and have difficulty sitting still very long. These symptoms are remarkably similar to children with autism and developmental disorders.

The use of midodrine in the treatment of adults with these autonomic symptoms often greatly improves their symptoms without causing excessive mental stimulation or exacerbation of their anxiety.

Midodrine works equally well in children. Midodrine is typically dosed first thing in the AM after waking with another dose midway between waking and going to bed for the night. This second dose is often around 1-3 PM.

The medication works within 25-30 minutes of the first dose so the positive effects can be immediately apparent. Because of the typical up-and-down variation in a child's behavior during the week, it might take a few days for the parents to appreciate its positive impact. Like all aspects of The Nemechek Protocol®, parental patience is key.

I often speak of midodrine as being a bridging therapy in that it is to be used for the limited amount of time between needing to better control the excessive behaviors and the time when the child recovers enough to be able to substantially control their own blood pressure and emotions without midodrine.

Midodrine also only works for about six hours so a parent only has to stop the medication on any given day to observe the child's behavior without the medication the following day.

The dose and use of midodrine are tapered as the autonomic nervous system recovers. Before discovering how to effectively get the autonomic nervous system to recover, I used midodrine often for adult patients with bothersome symptoms from low brain blood pressure. Now I rarely prescribe it and only for a short period because my patients often recover enough within a few months that it is no longer necessary.

Fight or Flight Versus Childhood Road Rage

In addition to properly regulating blood pressure, the ANS also influences how we regulate the intensity of our emotional response to certain situations to keep us safe. The ANS is constantly scanning the environment for cues of safety, danger, and life-threatening situations. This threat assessment and response system was coined "neuroception" by Dr. Stephen Porges and is a central tenet of his Polyvagal Theory.

When our ANS determines that our environment is safe, our defensive responses are suppressed, and we feel calm. When a threat or potential danger is perceived, the sympathetic branch of the ANS increases our sense of vigilance and will trigger protective responses that make the individual more aggressive and willing to fight or flee the from the perceived threat.

The threat assessment and response system operates below the radar of your awareness, but you can physically feel its presence. People often refer to this system when they describe an inner voice or their intuition about a situation that made them feel fearful. Injuries to the ANS can cause the threat assessment and response system to work incorrectly.

If the brain is unable to fully recover and cumulative brain injury occurs, consistent irregularities in a person's ability to properly perceive what is threatening and what is not will result in the brain not knowing how to properly respond to situations.

The term "road rage' is often used when discussing the excessive reaction of automobile drivers in stressful traffic situations. Road rage occurs when the threat assessment and response system has been damaged from a brain injury and causes individuals to overreact to perceived threats.

When working properly, the threat assessment and response system regulates the level of vigilance a person requires when driving. Whether they are driving on an isolated country road or a busy highway with highspeed traffic, the threat assessment and response system constantly monitors the potential danger of the present situation and forces the driver to apply the proper amount of vigilance to allow them to operate the automobile safely.

For example, on a country road a person may drive in a somewhat relaxed manner because they are traveling at lower speeds with little traffic and often plenty of visibility because of the wide-open spaces. But when driving at higher speeds on a highway, there is more danger and the driver's threat assessment and response system will increase their level of vigilance. Being more careful on a busy highway may seem like common sense but much of the increased vigilance one experiences when driving is subconsciously produced by the threat assessment and response system of the ANS.

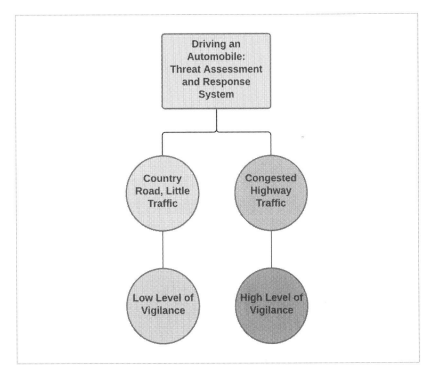

Threat Assessment and Response System of the ANS

A healthy ANS will not allow a person to drive in a casual, unsafe manner on a busy highway like they would on a country road. Driving casually on a busy highway is too dangerous, and the ANS is designed to protect them and keep them alive. The threat assessment and response system forces the driver to maintain their focus and vigilance by scanning traffic, keeping within a reasonably safe speed, and maintaining control of the steering wheel. Their vigilance increases as the intensity of the traffic increases. When somebody pulls in front of them in a potentially dangerous manner, their threat assessment and response system helps them to react quickly in order to avoid a collision. Importantly, as the external threat increases, the level of vigilance and heightened reaction also increases in an appropriate and measured manner.

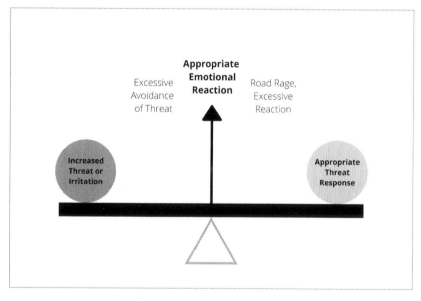

A Balanced Appropriate Emotional Reaction

Damage to the threat assessment and response system can prevent someone from being able to raise their vigilance enough such that they can no longer drive on the highway. Although they can handle the low-stress traffic of a country road or city street, their injury prevents them from increasing their vigilance enough to drive on the highway. I have seen this several times in adults who report that shortly after a trauma they inexplicably could not drive on the highway.

They feel as if some inner force prevents them from doing so because their anxiety levels would rise to intolerable levels if they drove on the highway. What they are reporting is that the damage they sustained from their brain injury has adversely affected their threat assessment and response system. Because of this injury, they are now incapable of increasing their threat management response to manage the potential threat of driving their automobile at higher speeds.

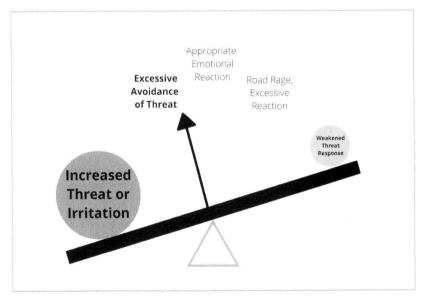

Excessive Avoidance of Threat

Sometimes injuries can have the opposite effect. Instead of not being able to increase the level of vigilance to match the stressful event, the threat assessment and response system over-responds and the driver demonstrates an excessively aggressive response commonly referred to as road rage.

The aggressive road rage behaviors occurs when another driver's behavior strikes the individual with a damaged threat assessment and response system as irritating or even dangerous. Their response to the event is excessive. Instead of simply feeling annoyed or frightened and trying to lessen the danger of the moment, the driver with road rage will have an excessive response that might involve yelling, aggressive gesturing, and might even chase the other driver.

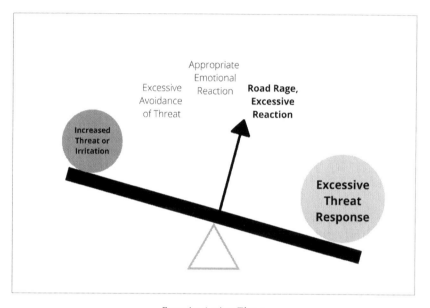

Excessive Against Threat

It often surprises people when I discuss road rage from an ANS damage perspective because road rage not an uncommon issue with my adult patients and most recover nicely with The Nemechek Protocol®. As the chronic damage to their nervous system is repaired, their anxiety or aggression when driving on the highway often dissipates.

Road Rage for Children

From a child's perspective, a threatening situation can arise when another child attempts to take their toy (conflict management), when there is an unanticipated change in the schedule of events (transition issues), or are given a command to do something they do not want to do (time to put the iPad away).

If their autonomic threat assessment and response system is working correctly, their reaction to these scenarios will be measured and appropriate. They follow the command but may pout or mildly show their displeasure but still follow through with the command.

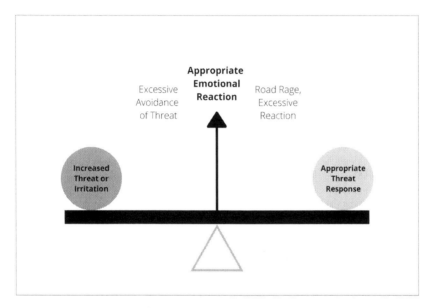

A Balanced Appropriate Emotional Reaction

But when the ANS is not working correctly because of a brain injury, the response to these situations can result in either an excessive avoidance response or an excessively aggressive response of the threat assessment and response system.

In children, a weakened management response to the potential threats might cause the child to retreat to a different room when strangers or even their own siblings enter the same room they presently occupy.

The child's retreat to a different room occurs because a prior injury to the threat assessment and response system cannot increase the level of vigilance to manage the complexity of the situation. This is a common response in children with autism and developmental disorders.

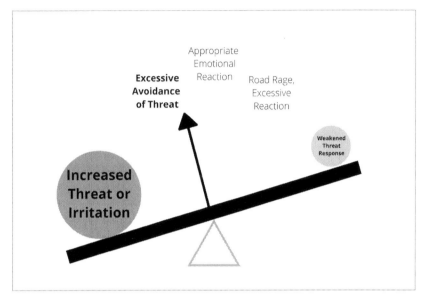

Excessive Avoidance of Threat

Occasionally the child's damaged threat assessment and response system will trigger an excessive response similar to road rage. When another person tries to take away an item the child is interested in at the moment (toy, iPad, etc.) or if there is a sudden change in the schedule or there is any request by a parent, therapist, or teacher that is not welcomed by the child, the child reacts with excessive aggression similar to road rage. Hair pulling, biting, scratching, kicking, and punching are the result of an excessive primitive response by the threat assessment and response system.

This reaction is often referred to as a problem with transitioning. Actually, I see it as road rage arising from an irritating situation because the aggression is not triggered if a child is transitioned to a favored activity such as receiving ice crease or a cookie.

This is not an unusual situation in some children with autism and/or developmental issues. Fortunately, the neurological damage leading to this response can recover with The Nemechek Protocol® just like it does in adults.

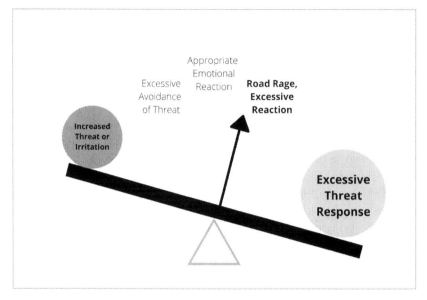

Excessive Against Threat

The aggressive behaviors may also be mislabeled as "defiance" as if the child has a willful, controllable role in the reaction. Behavior modification techniques are unsuccessful in controlling these reactions. These moments are not about the child's chosen desire to behave aggressively.

The reactions are an excessive, uncalibrated, aggressive biological response that is primitive and powerful, and that most children are incapable of controlling. The child wants to please their parents or therapists and certainly does not wish them harm. As most parents whose child behaves in such a manner, the children almost universally show remorse for the harm they may have caused someone.

These aggressive moments of road rage are very primitive in design and are being triggered at a subconscious level. The child has limited control over them and very often demonstrates remorse after their reaction harms another.

Identifying Road Rage from Low Blood Pressure Anxiety

In order to effectively manage the child's emotional ups and downs, its necessary to differentiate between the fight or flight reaction of low blood pressure from the aggressive responses of "road rage." Both involve a heightened emotional state with what can appear to be anxiety, aggression, or anger and can easily be confused with each other.

The protocol will help the autonomic nervous system to recover enough to allow both defects to substantially recover. Until that time, the difference in managing the events is quite different for the parent.

The low blood pressure event can be avoided or managed with increased fluid or salt intakes, moving the child into a horizontal position (laying down on the couch or the floor to read or play) or the use of midodrine to boost the blood pressure. If the anxious, aggressive event seems to be triggered without any irritant, this is likely a fight or flight reaction from excessively low brain blood pressure. These events might occur if the child is sitting in a chair or the car too long, has a mild infection, becomes too hot, or has not had enough to eat or drink recently. Kids with poor blood pressure regulation often are quite fidgety or hyperactive and seem to be frequently thirsty or hungry.

When an excessively aggressive response is triggered by phrases such as "time to put that away," "we can't (do what the child wants)," or "you are going to (the expected event)", this is likely a road rage response from a damaged threat assessment and response system. Road rage events might be managed with better transition planning, distraction from precipitating irritants or in the more severe cases behavior-modifying medications.

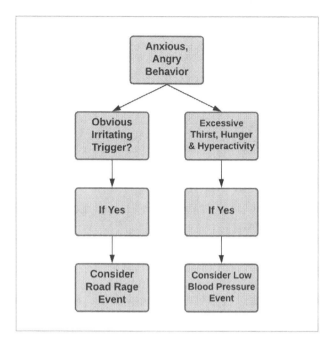

Low Blood Pressure vs. Road Rage

In my experience, it's not unusual for kids to have some features of both but the children with the most serious and even dangerous road rage events tend to do so in or approaching their teenage years.

Often, a child with autism and/or developmental issues will have a history of being hyperactive and frequently hungry or thirsty. The parents have become attune to managing this by keeping plenty of fluids or snacks handy, especially when traveling in order to keep their child's anxious tantrums under control. A slang term for this observation is "hangry," a combination of "the words hungry" and "angry." Then, as some children age, a different pattern of recognizable road rage aggression begins, often without any obvious cause to the parents.

The parents, therapists, and teachers often look for causes that would trigger excessive anger in a typically rational individual with a healthy, functioning threat assessment and response system. When they fail to find a reason, they often start talking about defiance issues with labels such as Oppositional Defiance Disorder.

They should instead be looking for a potentially traumatic event that damaged the autonomic threat assessment and response system.

Potential Traumas Leading to Road Rage

- **Physical Injury:** concussion or sub-concussive events

- **Inflammatory Injury:** surgery, vaccinations, fractures

- **Emotional Trauma:** moving to a new home, change in trusted therapist, bullying

When interviewing the parents about the time frame immediately prior to the onset of the road rage aggression, I can frequently identify potential emotional or physical traumas that potentially could have injured the autonomic nervous system further.

More often than not, it is the unavoidable emotional trauma that jumps out as a most likely cause. Some tantrums might be appropriate for the approximate maturity level of the child, but these tend to be rather self-limited, never aggressive, and have an obvious cause.

Regardless of the source of the trauma, The Nemechek Protocol® can help the child repair the damaged autonomic threat assessment and response system and the events will decrease and often ultimately cease altogether.

Management of Road Rage in a Child

After determining that the patient does indeed have the road rage type of aggressive episodes, I'll need to come up with a treatment plan to help minimize the events and help them recover as soon as possible before they cause serious injury to themselves or another person.

The first step is to start the child with excessive aggression issues on The Nemechek Protocol® . I including vagus nerve stimulation because it increases the chances that the child will have the broadest improvement of these potentially dangerous outbursts.

As the ANS recovers, the road rage aggression can lessen in intensity and the frequency of rage events can ultimately stop. The second step to avoiding or limiting the frequency of aggressive outbursts is to recognize that they do not come from willful, self-directed desires but rather from an involuntary impulse designed by evolution to help us survive.

The child's emotional responses are simply misfiring because of underlying autonomic damage. It is important to remember this is not from a lack of love or desire. They are simply not capable of the impulse control required to suppress these behaviors. Trying to reason with a developmentally handicapped child during an autonomic road rage event will often prove futile and frustrating for everyone. If you have ever been in an automobile with someone exhibiting road rage, you understand that rationalizing with them rarely ever has any impact on their impulsive behavior at that moment.

What is needed is a consistent, predictable schedule of events that is flexible from a time perspective and recognition that the child needs to be in a positive mindset for any necessary changes to the schedule. In other words, minimize the irritating moments of conflict as much as possible. A parent may plan a schedule for the day for the child in a way they can comprehend and post it somewhere that the child see it. If reading skills are lacking, consider using pictures or symbols to represent the activity instead of words and using pictures of school or mealtimes (breakfast, lunch, and dinner) as reference points instead of time. I know this isn't always practical, but I have learned from parents that this example is just one strategy to manage the environment of the child until such time that the protocol can sufficiently repair the threat assessment and response system and the excessive road rage behaviors cease to occur.

Finally, if the aggressive episodes are a dangerous threat to the child or those caring for them, prescription medications may be justified to control the dangerous behaviors. These medications should be prescribed under the guidance of a physician, and preferably one who understands the brain's responses to inadequate oxygen delivery from autonomic dysfunction. If they do not, find one who does or get them a copy of this book to read.

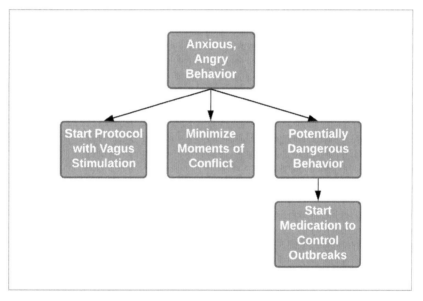

Managing Excessive Aggression

I have cared for children and young adults who were originally taking one or two potent, anti-psychotic medications to control their aggressive behavior and ultimately were able to wean off the medications without an increase in aggressive behavior within six to twelve months of starting the protocol. Weaning of any of these medications should be done with the guidance of the prescribing physician.

On occasion, these children and young adults will experience an increasing sense of self-awareness when the fight or flight and the road rage episodes from autonomic damage subside. Some have asked their parents, "What happened to me? How come I don't remember middle school?" Others will deny their prior behaviors occurred despite seeing video graphic evidence to the contrary.

Keep in mind the injured brain may not have been able to create memories from these past moments. This phenomenon is similar to what we witness in some of our recovering Alzheimer's patients who regain their sense of presence and self-awareness.

PART V

THE SCIENCE BEHIND THE NEMECHEK PROTOCOL®

14

SETTING THE STAGE FOR AUTISM - THE DETAILED VERSION

T his chapter will explain in greater detail some key concepts so you understand how we got to this modern-day health-care crisis, and why the components of The Nemechek Protocol® are effective when used consistently together.

Normal Brain Development

The Nemechek Protocol® can help many childhood issues such as autism, developmental disorders, ADD/ADHD and mood disorders because they all have the similar origin of overgrowth of intestinal bacteria and multiple mechanisms that fuel inflammation.

Normal brain development requires a healthy environment for the brain to develop fully and quickly and for a child to develop neuro-logically, they need to be able to prune neurons, repair brain injuries, and form neural networks.

As explained previously, a child is born with approximately one hundred billion neurons and they must trim these down to fifty billion neurons. The excess neurons provide developmental flexi-bility for the brain to acquire a new skill or ability. Most excess neurons are pruned away within the first five to six years of life.

Failure to trim the neurons fast enough is a major cause of developmental issues.

If the failure to trim is mild and the neurons simply are not being trimmed fast enough, we often refer to this as developmental delay. If the neuronal trimming process has severely slowed or even stopped completely, the child may be classified as having developmental arrest.

A common cause of altered neuronal pruning is from the impaired functioning of a specialized central nervous system white blood cell known as a microglia.

Microglia are referred to as the 'master gardener' because one of their primary roles is to tend to the neurons that branch throughout the brain like the branches of plants throughout a garden. Microglia tend to the neuron branches by either pruning them away like branches of a tree or by protecting and repairing them.

The initial distribution of neurons is somewhat random as the child's brain is having to discover a connection between bodily movements and brain function. The developmental process involves forming the pathways that will allow your child to track your face with their eyes or roll over in their crib. These behaviors occur only when the child's brain finds the neurons that connect the thought (follow the mother's face) to the action (move my eyes and head). Microglia sense these neuronal pathways are important and start nurturing and protecting them. If other neurons are not being used in any meaningful way, they will eventually be trimmed away as excess.

The process of pruning away the excessive neurons is necessary for the brain to survive. Neurons consume large amounts of energy. It is inefficient for the human body to spend energy on pathways that are not important for survival. At the time of birth, the brain consumes nearly 85% of all oxygen and calories but by the time a person reaches eighteen years of age it has been "pruned down" to an organ that only consumes 20% of all oxygen and calories. From an evolutionary viewpoint, this is a much more manageable percentage of energy consumption.

The neuronal pruning process continues throughout the child's life as they learn to crawl, stand upright, talk, walk, run, read, calculate, and mature into young adults. When children are running, playing, and mentally engaged in challenging activities, the pruning process is trying to refine the neurological pathways that support these activities. The microglia not only trim and maintain the normal sequence of maturation, but they also help repair the brain injuries that can occur from common physical (concussion and sub-concussive injuries), emotional (bullying, absence of a parent, intense fear, etc.), and inflammatory (surgery, fractures, vaccinations) traumas.

If the brain is being correctly pruned and repaired, then collections of neurons will begin to be formed as the child learns new skills, social behaviors, and life skills. These collections of neurons are referred to as neural networks. The formation of neural networks is what occurs when one learns to play the piano (or any other complex skill for that matter). Your understanding of music and the dexterity to play start slowly and one can only manage the simplest tune. This happens because a small grouping of neurons is connected in neural network. The neural network will expand by "crowd sourcing" more and more neurons as you learn to play more and more complex musical scores. It is the expanding number of neurons within the neural network that allows someone to ultimately play a very complex musical score such as Chopin on the piano.

Learning the social skills necessary to become a mature eighteen year old occurs in a similar fashion. Slowly over time, children learn to share, be patient, follow social rules expected from the family and community. Just as the skills required to play Chopin require many years, the development of neural networks for socialization will also require many years.

So collectively, children must be able to prune neurons, repair neurons and built neural networks in order to normally develop neurologically and form the complex neural networks required to function in society. What is happening globally now is that bacterial overgrowth within the small intestine can fully disrupt the process of neurological maturation.

This is not a temporary problem. Microglia function can be permanently and adversely altered by five different events all leading to a form of microglia that no longer prunes nor repairs the neurons.

5 Events That Trigger Primed Microglia

- Recurrent Concussions
- Encephalitis (severe brain infection)
- LSP leakage from Small Intestine Bacterial Overgrowth
- Chronic Inhalation of Microparticles from Diesel Exhaust
- Exposure to High Levels of Pro-Inflammatory Cytokines While in the Womb

Bacterial overgrowth, also known as SIBO (small intestine bacterial overgrowth), and the excessive concentration of bacteria overwhelms the integrity of the small intestine and leads to the leakage of lipopolysaccharide (LPS), a molecular component of a bacteria's outer shell and is only found on bacteria that live in the colon. A scientific term for the LPS-releasing bacteria is "gram-negative rod bacteria."

A study looking at overweight and obese children found that over 70% had evidence of SIBO. This is important in regard to autism as well as developmental disorders because the overgrowth of bacterial within the small intestine is the only known process that can both produce propionic acid as well as disrupt the normal pruning and repair process.

Bacterial Overgrowth Leads to Neurological Problems

Bacterial overgrowth is a condition where the person's normal intestinal bacteria end up living in the wrong place. They are not foreign or "bad" bacteria, these are bacteria that should normally live within the colon but now are in the upper or small intestine. Normally the species of bacteria living within the small intestine are different species from those living within the large intestine (also known as the colon).

As explained briefly in chapter 2, the two types of bacteria within the small and large intestine are so different from one another that its easiest to think of one type as birds (the normal residents of the small intestine) and the other type as fish (the normal residents of the colon).

Having a normal variety of bacterial species within the entire upper and lower intestinal tract is possibly the most important factor in preventing bacterial overgrowth. The bacterial themselves are actively involved in maintaining their separation. Studies of patients with recurrent bacterial overgrowth with *clostridium difficile* demonstrated that individuals with the lowest species counts are those most likely to have recurrent bacterial overgrowth. This is referred to as having low biodiversity of the intestinal microbiome.

Two other major factors that contribute to bacterial overgrowth include proper acidity of the small intestine as well as maintaining a normal level of forward intestinal propulsion or motility of the intestinal tract. Disruption of intestinal acidity with potent antacids and slowing of the forward propulsion that can occur after brain trauma, medications (anesthetics, pain medications), intestinal or abdominal surgery, or certain medical conditions (renal failure, scleroderma) are all well-documented triggers of intestinal bacterial overgrowth.

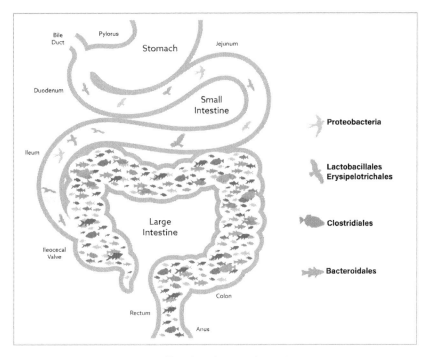

Normally Balanced intestinal Bacteria

There is an exceptionally large difference in the concentration of the number of bacteria that live within the small intestine as compared to the large intestine. For every individual "bird" bacterium in the upper small intestine, there is normally a hundred million "fish" bacteria living in the lowest portion of the colon; an enormous 1:100,000,000 difference in bacterial concentrations.

Bacterial intestinal overgrowth occurs when a single species of "fish" bacteria that normally live in the large intestine migrates upstream into the small intestinal tract and starts replicating out of control among the "bird" bacteria. Just as everyone understands that fish should not be living where birds live, large intestine bacteria should not be replicating in the small intestine where the "bird" bacteria live.

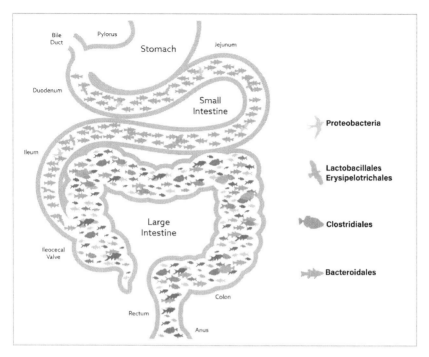

Bacterial Overgrowth of the Small Intestine (SIBO)

After the "fish" bacteria have migrated into the small intestine, there are not enough other bacteria to prevent them from growing out of control. Their overwhelming numbers overwhelm the design of the small intestine and allows the leakage of molecules into the surround tissue in a process known as bacterial translocation or "leaky gut." It is important to state that in spite of the common beliefs to the contrary, there is no scientific evidence that yeast, fungi, candida nor parasites cause "leaky gut." Leakage of molecules from digested food and bacterial cell walls can trigger the release of a very large amount pro-inflammatory cytokines throughout the body. The stress from these pro-inflammatory cytokines alter the normal function of cells throughout the body.

Bacterial translocation may also trigger the abnormal release of a wide variety of hormones, histamine, small chain fatty acids, and potential toxins. They can also trigger abnormal reactions to common foods (tomatoes, bananas, milk, citrus, etc.), causes skin reactions (psoriasis, rosacea, eczema, hives, rashes), and send signals to the brain potentially altering almost every aspect of brain, body, and cellular function.

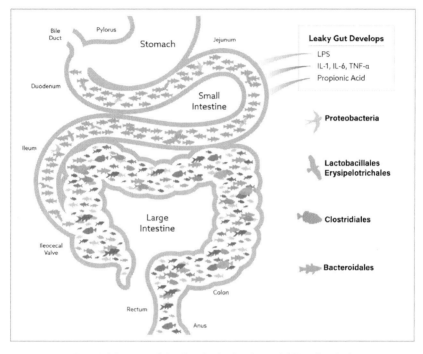

Bacterial Overgrowth Leads to Leaky Gut (Bacterial Translocation)

When bacterial translocation from overgrowth occurs fragments of the bacteria cell membrane called lipopolysaccharide (LPS) leaks into the bloodstream causing an exceptionally large release of pro-inflammatory cytokines and can permanently alter the function of a special white blood cell within the brain known as microglia.

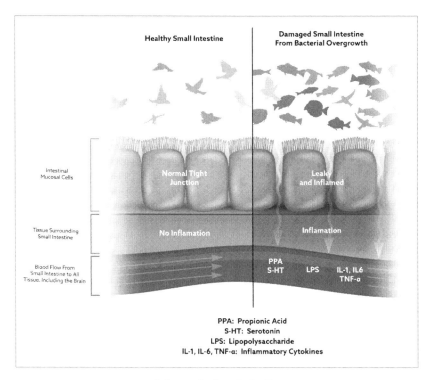

Healthy Small Intestine

Damaged Small Intestine
From Bacterial Overgrowth

Intestinal
Mucosal Cells

Normal Tight
Junction

Leaky
and Inflamed

Tissue Surrounding
Small Intestine

No Inflamation

Inflamation

Blood Flow From
Small Intestine to All
Tissue. Including the Brain

PPA
S-HT

LPS

IL-1, IL6
TNF-α

PPA: Propionic Acid
S-HT: Serotonin
LPS: Lipopolysaccharide
IL-1, IL-6, TNF-α: Inflammatory Cytokines

Inflammation from Leaky Gut

The altered microglia are called "primed MI-microglia" and their function changes from a helpful cell that prunes healthy neurons as well as repairs damaged neurons into a permanently inflammatory cell that prevents normal childhood development as well as magnifies the damage from common brain traumas.

If LPS priming and the release of pro-inflammatory cytokines occurs before the age of five or six, children will experience both developmental problems (delay of milestones, sensory issues, motor delay, intellectual delay), as well as manifest problems associated with poor repair of injuries (constipation, hyperactivity, poor focus, anxiety and aggression).

If LPS priming and the release of pro-inflammatory cytokines occurs after the age of 6 or so, the pruning of the brain will have been completed and so consequently there will be no evidence of developmental problems. The brain will still have difficulty repairing injuries and the children may experience attention issues (ADD), recurrent headaches, lightheadedness and passing out (syncope), constipation, abdominal cramping, reflux (GERD) and even premenstrual syndrome (PMS).

Other less common factors capable of triggering the primed M1-microglia include a serious brain infection referred to as encephalitis (e.g. Ebola, Dengue), a high frequency of concussions (e.g. American football or hockey), chronic exposure to diesel exhaust (e.g. living in the slums of highly polluted cities such as Beijing or Mexico City) and high levels of maternal inflammation during pregnancy of the child (i.e., mother is hospitalized with septic shock).

Common childhood injuries such as insignificant falls and bumps to the head that all children experience as they crawl, walk, play, interact with siblings, and explore their environment. We have all had a similar experience of a crying child at the family reunion or the park because they hit their head while playing. This is a normal type of injury that children used to fully recover from automatically. Children would cry for a while, be comforted, calm down, and then they would be fine. We understand now that these simple head injuries more than likely cause minor brain damage that will be fully repaired with healthy microglia.

Presently, the same minor injury is not fully repaired by the excessive pro-inflammatory cytokines and primed M1-microglia that are triggered by bacterial overgrowth. Instead of recovering fully, the child is left with residual damage that grows overtime in a process referred to as cumulative brain injury.

One Hundred Years of Intestinal Bacterial Damage

In the womb, a child's intestinal tract contains little to no bacteria. It is only after birth that a child's intestinal tract becomes fully colonized from bacteria inhabiting the mother's intestinal tract. The two factors that are most important in the complete transmission of the mother's intestinal bacteria to her child are vaginal delivery and breastfeeding.

Studies suggest that humans were successfully passing the same blend of intestinal bacteria from mother to child for at least three million years. The only present-day individuals with relatively normal blends of intestinal bacteria consist of a few very primitive tribes (Yanomami, Guahibo Amerindians, Malawians, and African hunter-gatherers) and the loss of intestinal bacteria is believed to have begun around the turn of the last century.

Since the turn of the last century, each sequential maternal generation had their intestinal bacterial blend damaged in unique ways, compounding the previously damaged bacteria blend they received from their mother at birth. By examining the bacteria contained within the intestinal tracts of the entombed royalty of Genoa, Italy, stool specimens from ancient tombs as well as 1,000-year-old frozen humans discovered in glaciers, scientists have determined that the human biome has had the same mixture of bacterial species until around 1900. From this point forward it seems that every maternal generation has potentially lost of their bacterial species due to exposure to pesticides, antibiotics, and other chemicals. The damage to our intestinal microbiome has probably accelerated in the last 50 years as more and more potent antibiotics have been developed and commonly used for otherwise routine, minor infections.

Additionally, a child is born by caesarian section (c-section) and/or is bottle-fed, the mother's microbiome will not be fully transferred to her infant child and long-lasting differences between the child's and mother's intestinal bacteria can occur. If the mother's bacterial blend is already somewhat depleted prior to delivery, the child's bacterial blend may be depleted even further if born by cesarean section or if they are solely bottle-fed.

The bacterial issue is not just a mother-child issue. Both parents may contribute to the likelihood of bacterial overgrowth occurring and to its potential impact on the health of the child. Which bacteria may overgrow the small intestine, or what those bacteria might do once they overgrow, might be determined by genes contributed by the father as well as the mother. It is a complex combination of the mother's bacterial blend and genes from both parents as well as a multitude of life events after birth (antibiotic exposure, probiotics, diet, environmental chemicals, injury, surgery, food preservatives, and other unknown factors) that may result in an unhealthy blend of intestinal bacteria and the development of bacterial overgrowth.

At present most individuals have less than normal numbers of intestinal bacterial species after being born compared to people over one hundred years ago. This is referred to as having decreased microbiome diversity. As the number of unique species decreases further and further with each maternal generation, the bacteria seem to have less capacity to maintain the normal separation of the different bacteria within the small and large intestine.

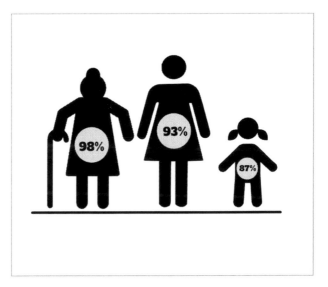

Decreasing Generational Microbiome Diversity

The decreased capacity to maintain the intestinal balance is compounded further when the function of the intestinal tract is further altered from brain trauma, intestinal infections, antibiotics, vaccines, antacids (proton pump inhibitors), probiotics, general anesthesia, abdominal surgery and other medical procedures.

The collective effect of low biodiversity and these other factors creates an increased likelihood of children and adults developing small intestine bacterial overgrowth (SIBO). Once overgrowth occurs, the small intestine is unable to withstand the stress of the increased bacterial load. Small molecules from bacterial cell walls and food particles are then capable of leaking into the surrounding tissue in a process referred to as bacterial translocation or "leaky gut." Bacterial translocation can trigger a surge of pro-inflammatory cytokines. Eighty percent of the entire immune system, including white blood cells and mast cells, are in the tissues immediately surround the small intestine.

In additional, highly inflammatory molecules such as LPS may escape into the blood stream, enter the central nervous system, and alter the normal function of microglia within the brain. As discussed in this chapter, microglia are instrumental in the process of pruning neurons in children as well as repairing the neurons in both children and adults. Once exposed to LPS, the microglia become permanently inflammatory and their pruning and repairing of neurons stops altogether.

However, the behavior of primed M1-microglia can be normalized with a wide variety of experimental chemical compounds and devices. This change in the behavior of microglia is referred to as phenotypic shifting. The Nemechek Protocol® has been designed to prevent primed M1-microglia from causing further damage. The use of vagus nerve stimulation, high concentrations of the omega-3 fatty acid DHA, and extra virgin olive oil have been shown in animal models to cause primed M1-microglia to shift their behavior into an anti-inflammatory, tissue-repairing M2-microglia. Not all children are destined to develop bacterial overgrowth even if they have low biodiversity of their intestinal bacteria. If bacterial overgrowth never occurs, their neurological development and recovery from brain traumas should continue normally.

Pointers on helping maintain a healthy balance of bacteria is an otherwise healthy child is provided in the chapter on prevention.

Primed M1-Microglia Magnify Brain Injury

The unregulated and permanent inflammatory behavior of primed M1-microglia magnify the degree of damage caused by common brain injuries and prevent stem cells and other repair mechanisms (neurotrophins) from repairing the damage that would have fully recovered with normal functioning microglia.

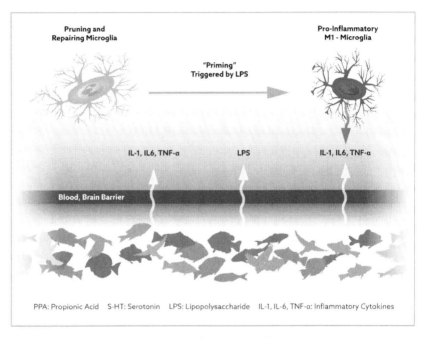

Triggering of Primed Microglia

The impairment of microglia may also be responsible for the abnormal white matter structure within the brain that seems to be associated with sensory perception disorders.

The magnified damage and incomplete recovery caused by primed M1-microglia are the hallmark features of a pathological process called cumulative brain injury or CBI.

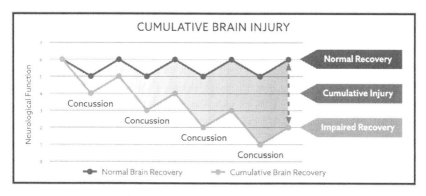

Cumulative Brain Injury from Physical Brain Trauma

Cumulative brain injury from primed M1-microglia is occurring in an epidemic fashion throughout the population and is the predominant feature behind the well-publicized problems of professional football players contracting chronic traumatic encephalopathy (CTE).

Cumulative brain injury develops not only from physical injuries, but can occur from emotional trauma and the release of high levels of pro-inflammatory cytokines from surgery or fractures of large bones, as well as vaccinations.

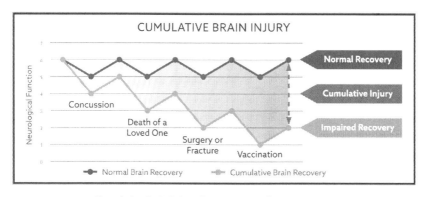

Cumulative Brain Injury from a Variety of Brain Traumas

In addition to primed M1-microglia not pruning neurons correctly and causing varying degrees of developmental delay, the cumulative brain injury effect from primed microglia is also allowing small brain injuries to stack upon previously unresolved brain injuries.

Cumulative brain injury from primed M1-microglia is also a suspected factor in the development of attention deficit/hyperactivity disorder (ADD/ADHD), epilepsy, Alzheimer's dementia, Parkinson's disease, chronic depression, bipolar disorder, schizophrenia, and post-traumatic stress disorder.

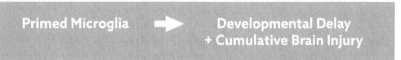

Primed Microglia ➡ Developmental Delay + Cumulative Brain Injury

When bacterial overgrowth occurs, it will trigger developmental delay which can range from mild to severe. In addition to developmental delay, the child may also accumulate damage via CBI to the autonomic nervous system.

A dysfunctional autonomic nervous system is responsible for many common childhood problems such as constipation, IBS, reflux, ADD, ADHD, fidgety movements, toe-walking, headaches, persistent hunger as well as anxiety.

The increase of inflammation released from primed M1-microglia and the intestinal tract have the potential to lower the seizure threshold and increase both the likelihood and the frequency of epileptic seizures. This effect is often seen in children younger than one year of age as febrile seizures, its most benign form.A febrile seizure is a relatively harmless event in very young children that lasts less than a minute and occurs when the child is running a temperature. This is an "out of the blue" event in an otherwise healthy child. In this situation, the child develops an inflammatory response and a fever after contracting a common viral infection. The inflammation then lowers the seizure threshold causing the child to have a seizure. These seizures do not return unless the fever and inflammatory reaction occur again. Fortunately, children usually grow out of this pattern by their first birthday once their nervous system matures further.

Increased Inflammation ➡ Increased Chance of Seizure

Once bacterial overgrowth occurs in the child, the cascade of LPS leakage, microglia priming, failure of neuronal pruning, and increased pro-inflammatory cytokine levels has now set the stage for developmental delay and cumulative brain injury, so now all it takes is one more pathological twist and autism occurs.

The feature that turns a child with developmental delay, ADD, headaches, and anxiety into a child who develops autism is the over-production of a short-chain fatty acid called propionic acid by colonic bacteria which are now replicating out of control within the small intestine.

15

SLIPPING INTO AUTISM

The Sedating Effect of Propionic Acid

T here are many, many different bacterial species within the large intestine that can potentially flux up into the small intestine and begin growing in excess. When bacterial over-growth occurs within the small intestine, it is typically from a single species of bacteria.

Some bacteria are capable of producing propionic acid while others are not. Many of these are propionic-producing bacteria from the clostridium family and when they are given the opportunity to grow out of control within the small intestine, a large amount of propionic acid is produced and absorbed into the bloodstream. When propionic acid levels rise in the bloodstream, laboratory animals begin behaving strangely as if intoxicated. The same effect seems to be occurring in children when their intestinal tract is overgrown with enough propionic acid-producing bacteria. The stuporous, drug-like effect of propionic acid is the primary cause of "loss of eye contact and awareness" when autism is first noted.

Children may be developing normally and it is only after an event (course of antibiotics, a surgical procedure, a strong antacid, or a vaccination) triggers bacterial overgrowth with a propionic acid producing bacterial species that the parents will see a sudden shift in their child's demeanor and behavior. The sudden change in the child's behavior is because they are intoxicated with propionic acid. The medical term for this is toxic encephalopathy.

The transition into autism begins whenever the propionic acid production levels are high enough to saturate the brain of the child and begin altering the child's behavior. The timing of that increase of propionic acid explains why many parents report they observed their child change before their eyes while other parents report their child demonstrated autistic and other developmental features since birth. In other cases, parents report a slow transition into this drugged state over several months.

Although a newborn child adopts their mother's intestinal bacterial blend at birth, many other factors are often involved for the child to slip into autism. Those other factors influencing the child's bacterial blend could include genetic abnormalities, a stay in the neonatal intensive care unit (NICU), the use of potent antacids referred to as proton pump inhibitors, general anesthesia, a surgical procedure to repair a hole in the heart, or pyloric stenosis, or the mother requiring IV antibiotics just prior to delivery.

A child's father can also contribute to the child's risk of developing autism by contributing genes that might (1) increase the risk of bacterial overgrowth in general (2) favor the overgrowth of the propionic-producing bacteria versus non-propionic acid producing bacteria, or (3) cause microglia to be more sensitive to the priming effects of LPS thereby being more apt to cause developmental delay or cumulative brain injury with low levels of bacterial overgrowth and LPS exposure.

Autism = Mother (propionic producing bacterial
overgrowth + genes)
+ Father (genes)
+ Other Events

The primary pathophysiological difference between a child with developmental issues and ADD, when compared to a child with autism, developmental issues and ADD, is the production of large quantities of propionic acid. And the difference between both of those examples when compared to a child with no evidence of autism, developmental delay, or any effects of cumulative brain injury (ADD, anxiety, or headaches), is a normally balanced intestine tract.

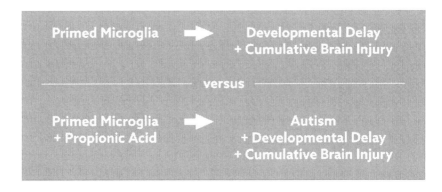

Once the bacterial overgrowth is reversed and propionic acid levels decline, the children are released from the toxic, stuporous prison they have been trapped in. This is what I previously called "the awakening" period. During this awakening period, children will have improved eye contact and become more aware of their surroundings. The awakening may manifest as being more observant of their environment, more interactive, and more calm. The awakening period is more pronounced in younger children with autism and often is not as apparent in teenagers and young adults with autism.

On the other hand, some children in the awakening period will demonstrate a greater level of anxiety, hyperactivity, aggression, hunger, thirst, and insomnia. These heightened and potentially disruptive behaviors are usually the manifestation of the child's underlying neurological impairment that was not previously as apparent because of the powerful sedating effects of propionic acid. Similar to a powerful pharmaceutical sedative, once the propionic acid levels dissipate, the aberrant behaviors will become apparent.

Another cause of disruptive behaviors in some children is when excessive doses of inulin are used to balance the intestinal tract. As the inulin dose is increased, a child might become more anxious, hyperactive, hungry, thirsty or aggressive. Their increasingly disruptive behavior mimics what is seen in adults when their brain blood pressure is suboptimal and is referred to as cerebral hypoperfusion.

In adults, cerebral hypoperfusion often is the result of autonomic nervous system dysfunction and commonly leads to anxiety, poor focus, increase hunger and/or thirst, fidgety behaviors, and insomnia. Adults will report that all of these symptoms improve if they improve brain blood pressure by exercising, eating carbohydrates or salt, drinking fluids or simply lying flat. All of these behaviors increase blood flow to the brain.

Children experiencing low blood pressure react in the same manner. They will constantly be hungry or thirsty, frequently lay flat on the sofa or floor, sometimes hang their head over the edge of the bed, toe walk and have such an urge to move their muscles they are hyperactive.

Their young brain has a remarkable capacity to begin trimming neurons so they can catch up developmentally, as well as repair the underlying cumulative damage from past injuries. Post injury studies show that the brain can produce new neurons at the site of injury as well as have neurons migrate to different areas of the brain where they are needed.

I like to say the process of catching up developmentally and repairing underlying brain injury is like watching your hair grow, it is a slow but steady process. Day by day imperceptible recovery occurs, but before you know it, a new behavior or a milestone is gained. These new skills and improved behaviors will ebb and flow but always continue to grow in frequency and complexity.

I constantly remind parents that neurological recovery is a slow process and they must be patient. The gains frequently seen with The Nemechek Protocol® are often breathtaking and unparalleled but can take many months and even years to be fully realized.

We are in completely uncharted territory because the scope of this recovery has proven many theories about the impossibility of neurological recovery completely wrong.

In the future, I believe we will discover that bacterial overgrowth is responsible for the production of a variety of other toxic compounds other than propionic acid that contribute to a wide array of particular symptoms and illnesses in children as well as adults.

Potential examples I have seen in my patients is their recovery from stuttering, intense anxiety, insomnia, migraine headaches, dyslexia, tics, Tourette's and chronic hiccups that begin within a few weeks after restoring intestinal bacteria balance. Each of these disorders could potentially be triggered by an unusual chemical produced by a unique strain of overgrown bacteria.

Inflammation and Genetic Abnormalities

It is quite clear that autism and other pervasive developmental disorders are increasing in incidence and the wide variety of genetic mutations in 5-10% of cases may have an impact on the features of these disorders. While some autism genes have an obvious functional significance (SHANKs, neuroligins, and neurexins, fragile x syndrome, mental retardation-associated proteins), many autism genes do not present a clear mechanism of dysfunction. The clinical significance of these non-associated genes has yet to be determined.

When speaking of the impact of genetics concerning any medical disorder that is increasing in frequency, one must try to understand whether these genes are new within in the affected individual (such as can happen with radiation exposure, drug exposure during pregnancy, or even after birth) or whether the genes were pre-existing but dormant, in the parent from whom they were passed. Inflammation may play a role in both dormant and active genes. Elevated levels of pro-inflammatory cytokines are capable of activating genes that have laid dormant in preceding generations and trigger an illness associated with the gene.

Alternatively, pro-inflammatory cytokines may suppress genes that are needed to remain healthy and can oppositely lead to a medical condition.

Systemic inflammation also impairs the ability of stem cells and neurons to mature properly and may cause DNA to be miscopied (genetic 'typos') especially when the child is developing within the womb. This would result in the development of an abnormal cellular gene within the child that was not passed from either parent.

In either scenario, it is more than likely that previous generations did not have such a high prevalence of autism as we do today because they had healthier blends of intestinal bacteria and lived in an environment that produced much less systemic inflammation in their bodies.

Before birth, inflammatory cytokines are capable of causing mutations or activating/suppressing pre-existent genes present within the mother's body and this can influence the development or activation of the unborn child's cellular DNA.

Sources of Chronic Inflammation During Pregnancy

- Primed CNS (Central Nervous System) Microglia from Bacterial Overgrowth
- Deficient Dietary Omega-3 Fatty Acid Intake
- Excess Dietary Omega-6 Fatty Acids Intake
- Damage to the Autonomic Nervous System and the Vagus Inflammatory Reflex
- Excessive Ingestion of Saturated Fatty Acids
- Excessive Ingestion of Processed Carbohydrates
- Ingestion of Advanced Glycation End Products
- First or Second-Hand Tobacco Exposure
- Autoimmune Disorders
- Probiotic Use

This is an extensive list of sources of metabolic inflammation but the top four are the most common factors that seem to affect the health of the patients, both young and old, that I see in my practice.

The reduction of those sources of inflammation within both children and pregnant mothers may serve two distinct purposes regarding the development of autism. In pregnant mothers, less systemic inflammation will allow neuronal stem cells to develop correctly and would therefore lessen the likelihood of genetic-based medical disorders being triggered. In children, less systemic inflammation will allow microglia and cellular repair mechanisms to function more normally and effectively, thereby supporting a natural neuronal pruning process and a normal pace of development. Significant reductions of inflammation within the child may also allow unhealthy genes to be essentially switched off, resulting in no more harm to the individual, creating a remission state of a genetic disorder.

16

THE INFLAMMATORY-NEUROTOXIC
SPECTRUM

Historically, when scientists have tried to understand certain abnormal behaviors in individuals, they will group patients together under a certain heading based on the particular abnormal behavior observed by the researchers. Their approach is not much different than trying to figure out a 1,000-piece jigsaw puzzle.

Most of us will begin to organize the puzzle pieces according to certain characteristics such as a particular color, patterns, or pieces than encompass the flat edges of the puzzle.

Doing this helps us to make sense of a wide variety of seemingly unrelated pieces. Medical examples of the jigsaw puzzle approach based on observed, abnormal emotional behavior are depression, anxiety, schizophrenia, psychosis, and personality disorders.

Another grouping based on observed characteristics is the developmental disorders that affect children.

Developmental Diagnosis are Based on Observed Behaviors

The developmental jigsaw puzzle consists of observed autism spectrum disorders (autism, Asperger syndrome, or Pervasive Developmental Disorder-Not Otherwise Specified), pervasive developmental disorders (delays in the development of multiple basic functions), specific developmental disorders (delays in only a specific area), and other neurodevelopmental disorders such as traumatic brain injury (TBI), and attention deficit disorders (ADD, ADHD).

Developmental Disorder Spectrum

Autism Spectrum Disorder
Pervasive Developmental Disorder
Specific Developmental Disorder
Other Developmental Disorders (TBI, ADD, ADHD)

This system works well in the respect that a wide variety of research has shown that this particular treatment approach may help one aspect of a developmental disorder more than another. It also serves as a platform to help manage the distribution of supportive resources (therapists, medical care, school assistance, etc.) more efficiently.

The problem is that this observed organizational approach is not useful when trying to understand the underlying cause of these childhood disorders.

A Common Pathological Process for Many Developmental Disorders

Studies are outlining a process in which abnormally functioning microglia (a white blood cell) and elevated levels of pro-inflammatory cytokines within the central nervous system play a combined role in a wide range of neurological disorders in both adults and children.

In adults, the abnormal activation of microglia and elevated cytokines are associated with the development of Alzheimer's dementia, Parkinson's disease, amyotrophic lateral sclerosis (ALS), macular degeneration, treatment-resistant epilepsy, chronic depression, schizophrenia, post-traumatic stress disorder, post-concussion syndrome, as well as chronic traumatic encephalopathy (CTE) in athletes.

In children, this same pathological process is associated with impaired development of fundamental brain architecture, neuron migration, and synaptic pruning all leading to a variety of developmental issues, and the incomplete recovery from physical, emotional, and inflammatory brain trauma resulting in cumulative brain injury.

Therefore, to clearly understand how a single approach can positively affect so many seemingly different forms of childhood developmental issues, the approach needs to be viewed from the common pathway of microglia activation and pro-inflammatory cytokines.

I refer to this viewpoint as the inflammatory-neurotoxic spectrum of developmental disorders.

The Inflammatory-Neurotoxic Spectrum of Developmental Disorders

Instead of viewing developmental disorders from the perspective of the child's observed behavior, a clearer picture of the disease process is gained by viewing the disease process from a cellular pathological process. The variety of abnormal behavioral patterns reflects the variety of different areas of the brain that are not functioning correctly.

The concept is no different than observing the variety of manners in which a stroke may affect an adult. Some adults with a stroke may have paralysis of both their right arm and leg, others may have weakness in the left arm and are unable to speak or swallow, while others may simply begin to manifest dementia without any motor or sensory impairment of their limbs.

Each of these patterns of altered neurological function represents a different area of the brain that is affected by a similar pathological process. The same holds true for children with developmental disorders.

The wide variation of speech, sensory, motor, cognition, and emotional difficulties a child may experience simply represents the summation of different areas of their brain not working correctly.

The chronic brain dysfunction in children with developmental disorders occurs primarily through three different pathological processes which are:

- Unrepaired brain trauma resulting in cumulative brain injury
- Slow or abnormal neuronal pruning resulting in developmental delay
- Excessive production of propionic acid toxicity resulting in toxic encephalopathy

The degree or extent of developmental delay and cumulative brain injury are magnified with increasing levels of systemic and central nervous system pro-inflammatory cytokines coming from a variety of sources with the bacterial overgrowth of the small intestine contributing the most.

Bacterial overgrowth also contributes to the production of propionic acid capable of exerting a toxic effect on brain function in a fashion similar to a sedative such as Valium® (diazepam) or a hallucinogen such as LSD (lysergic acid diethylamide).

The Timing of Bacterial Overgrowth Determines if Cumulative Brain Injury Occurs With or Without Developmental Delay

A major determinant whether a patient's bacterial overgrowth results in simple cumulative brain injury symptoms such as constipation, or poor focus or results in developmental delay with possible autism is dependent on two factors – the age at which bacterial overgrowth first appears and whether or not the bacteria overgrowing in the small intestine are capable of producing propionic acid.

Since most neuronal pruning is completed by the time kids are five or six years old, the development of bacterial overgrowth before or after this age results in significant differences in the child. If a child has normal intestinal bacterial balance the first eight years of life, their microglia will be functioning normally, and they will be able to correctly prune and repair their nervous system avoiding any developmental or cumulative brain injury issues.

But if a child develops bacterial overgrowth at the age of eight, they will still not have any developmental issues but from this point forward they will have difficulty repairing traumas and over the ensuing years, the child might develop ADD, anxiety, and increasing constipation. All signs of cumulative brain injury.

If the same child develops bacterial overgrowth at the age of eight months instead of eight years, both normal pruning and normal repair processes will be affected. The child will develop neurological problems consistent with both developmental delays as well as cumulative brain injury.

At this point, the child may have impairment from developmental delay and cumulative brain injury, but these two factors are not enough to produce autism. The unique features attributed to autism require the bacteria to also produce large amounts of propionic acids.

Of the single species of bacteria that may overgrow within the small intestine, some do and some do not produce propionic acid. If they do produce propionic acid, you have autism with underlying developmental delay and cumulative brain injury. If they do not produce propionic acid, the patient will only have developmental delay and cumulative brain injury but no diagnosis of autism.

You can see that there can be three very different outcomes just based on the timing of when bacterial overgrowth occurs and if the bacteria do or do not produce large amounts of propionic acid.

Targeting Treatment for Autism and Developmental Disorders

Viewing developmental disorders of childhood through the lens of inflammation and propionic acid toxicity helps to explain how such a simple treatment regimen as The Nemechek Protocol® may affect so many seemingly different disorders.

The fact is that the primary underlying process that triggers most of these disorders is one and the same—bacterial overgrowth of the small intestine. The childhood disorders differ only with respect to the age at which bacterial overgrowth occurs, what area of the brain is not being pruned or repaired correctly, and whether the overgrowth bacteria are producing excessive propionic acid.

My model for autism is best understood as a theoretical model that is based on a wide variety of animal and human-based research. The "proof" for this model being correct in large part is that using it as a guide for treatment seems to be highly effective. To become more definitive, large studies are needed but no one is considering such a trial at the present, especially for something as inexpensive and accessible as fish oil, olive oil, and inulin (or rifaximin).

One thing is for sure: my simple approach to inflammation and propionic acid suppression is having an unprecedented positive effect on many children and adults around the world.

17

UNDERSTANDING HOW THE PROTOCOL WORKS IN 3 STEPS

Step One: Rebalancing the Intestinal Tract

Since developmental impairment and cumulative brain injury are fueled by the excessive production of pro-inflammatory cytokines and the core pathophysiological factor of autism is the production of propionic acid from bacterial overgrowth, establishing control over bacterial overgrowth is the most critical step of The Nemechek Protocol.

Some children and adults with intestinal bacterial overgrowth will show signs or symptoms of the overgrowth. Common symptoms of bacterial overgrowth include reflux or heartburn, specific food intolerance (tomatoes, spices, citrus, coffee, chocolate, etc.), watery or urgent stool, anxiety, or eczema.

It is not unusual for a child or an adult with bacterial overgrowth to not have any particular intestinal symptoms. Approximately 20-30 % of adults with intestinal bacterial overgrowth have no obvious intestinal symptoms.

Although there may be no noticeable intestinal symptoms, bacterial overgrowth is still capable of producing toxic levels of propionic acid and preventing both neuronal pruning and brain injury repair through elevated brain inflammation and abnormal microglia function. Because of these reasons, I believe all children with any aspect of autism or developmental issues need treatment to address small intestine bacterial overgrowth.

Preferred Method to Balance Intestinal Bacteria in Younger Children:

Inulin Prebiotic Fiber Supplementation
1/8 -1/2 teaspoon of inulin powder, 1 time per day

Inulin is an over the counter (OTC) prebiotic fiber that comes from a variety of natural plant sources. Inulin derived from agave, chicory root, and Jerusalem artichoke are all acceptable forms of inulin. Inulin prebiotic powder is inexpensive and is sold by a variety of manufacturers.

If the child is under eight years of age, I always start with inulin to balance intestine bacteria. If the child is between eight and fourteen, I start with either inulin or rifaximin.

I recommend giving my patients 1/8 to 1/2 teaspoon of inulin powder, once daily. It has been my experience that some children may go through some fluctuation of behavior or intestinal function for a week or two after starting the inulin fiber.

Beyond the dose of 1/2 teaspoons a day, it is rare to see any added improvement in symptoms and the higher dose has the potential to increase hyperactivity, hunger, thirst, anxiety, or aggression and may cause discomfort from excessive gas, cramping, or bloating.

Inulin powder is odorless and has a slightly sweet taste. Inulin powder may be taken with or without food and it may be mixed with hot or cold liquids of solids. Inulin is the only prebiotic fiber that I use with my patients.

Over the years I have tried different prebiotic fibers in my office but none of them reduced bacterial overgrowth enough to allowed brain recovery to occur in children and some fibers such as guar gum can potentially cause dangerous intestinal obstruction.

Inulin increases the acidity of the small intestine which results in suppressed growth of the colonic bacteria within the small intestine. When the growth of the colonic bacteria is suppressed, propionic acid production is dramatically reduced.

Propionic acid is a chemical compound that our bodies naturally produce so it is not something that we can completely stop, but it is something that can be reduced by controlling excessive bacterial overgrowth. Propionic acid is sometimes used as an additive in foods, but these amounts are so small that I do not believe they need to be avoided.

Prebiotic fibers are quite different from probiotic bacteria. Inulin is *not* a probiotic and inulin should *not* be used with a probiotic. All of my patients are instructed to immediately stop the use of all probiotics before starting The Nemechek Protocol®.

In an earlier chapter, I explained how the bacteria in the small intestine are so different from the bacteria living down in the colon that you could think of one type of them as birds (small intestine bacteria) and the other type as fish (colon bacteria).

Using the birds and fish illustration of SIBO, inulin fiber is best thought of as food for the healthy "bird" bacterial within the small intestine: inulin feeds the birds (the beneficial bacteria that should be there) but does not feed the fish (the invading bacteria). Inulin powder also comes in the form of chewable gummies. It has been my experience that one to two inulin gummies per day are enough to balance the intestinal tract in young children.

It has been my experience that some children seem to react negatively to dyes or other ingredients in a gummy, so if the patient seems to have a reaction, I switch them to pure inulin powder.

After starting the child on daily inulin, fish oil, and olive oil, parents often ask how they will know whether this is the right amount of inulin and fish oil for their young child. The first treatment goal is determine if the inulin is effective in reversing bacterial overgrowth with inulin or rifaximin might be necessary.

Determining if Inulin is Effective

Reversal of bacterial overgrowth with inulin will lead to a drop in propionic acid and often results in what I refer to as the awakening, especially in younger patients. The awakening occurs within the first 1-2 weeks and is manifested by the children showing more eye contact, more alertness, more engagement, and possibly even more stimming or insomnia.

Once the awakening occurs, the dose of inulin used is adequate because the sudden improvement in the child's behavior is evidence that the bacteria have been suppressed. No further increases in inulin dosage are necessary if the awakening occurs.

If the dosage of inulin is increased very, very slowly or the children are older, their awakening behaviors change so slowly that they are not noticed in spite of propionic acid being suppressed.

Improvements in neurological development will begin to occur at an increased pace over the following three-six months. If there is no significant improvement after three months, then the child is experiencing inulin failure and will need to be treated with rifaximin.

Pointers and FAQ's:

What type of inulin do I prefer? I prefer pure inulin powder for children (inulin is not very effective at controlling bacterial overgrowth in older teens and adults). When buying powdered inulin, I recommend buying Nemechek Blue Organic Inulin or Inulin from NOW Foods. It is my experience that many other brands are much less effective than

Nemechek Blue or the NOW Foods brand. A list of Nemechek-approved brands is listed in the appendix.

When might my patients first respond to treatment? Depending on the child's amount of underlying developmental delay, children may start making eye contact, becoming more aware of their surroundings, allowing more physical contact, or otherwise communicating and speaking more within a few days to weeks.

How fast of a pace might recovery occur?

Some studies indicate that developmental delay recovers at about a rate of two to three months for every calendar month that brain inflammation is lowered. Some children may recover this fast while other children take considerably longer. No matter the age of the child, the most important factor to consider is whether the protocol has increased the rate of improvement compared to the pace of any gains prior to the protocol.

How long do my patients need to stay on inulin and the rest of The Nemechek Protocol®? Propionic acid control and brain recovery are long term processes and each aspect of the protocol (intestinal balance, olive oil, and fish oil) have different timelines. Since we still do not understand how to completely prevent bacterial overgrowth from occurring, there will be an ongoing need to maintain the intestinal balance and reverse overgrowth should it occur.

The deficiency of omega-3 fatty acids and excess of omega-6 fatty acids within the food supply make the regular supplementation with omega-3 fatty acids from fish oil (at present) and olive oil a long-term health requirement.

Have I seen intestinal symptoms change after starting inulin?

Sometimes a patient's constipation or bloating seems to get worse after starting inulin. Constipation, heartburn, and bloating are signs of their underlying autonomic dysfunction and not a direct consequence of inulin. These only seem to "worsen" because inulin stops the watery or frequent stools associated with bacterial overgrowth and allows the underlying constipation or bloating to be more apparent.

Constipation and bloating will eventually resolve as The Nemechek Protocol® continues to improve autonomic function. If the child is uncomfortable or experiencing pain from constipation, I often recommend a non-fiber, non-digestive enzyme supplement such as magnesium (milk of magnesia) or MiraLAX®.

If the child is not having daily bowel movements but is comfortable and without pain, I recommend using these products only as needed and not to simply create a bowel movement daily.

What if the inulin worsens stimming?

If there seems to be excessive stimming after starting the inulin, I will recommend decreasing the inulin dose by an 1/8-1/4 of a tsp per day and see if things improve. It can sometimes take a week or two before the dosage reduction results in improved behaviors.

What if the child is having painful cramping or mucous in stool?

If the child is experiencing cramping or mucous in stool, I recommend the parents stop the use of any probiotics, digestive enzymes, or supplements. If these additional supplements are not being used, I recommend stopping the inulin for a week and then restarting it at a lower dose. If the symptoms still do not stop, I recommend having the child's pediatrican evaluate the child.

What if the child cannot tolerate inulin?

If a child is unable to tolerate inulin, then I recommend using a course of the prescription rifaximin to balance the intestinal tract.

What about other products for bacterial overgrowth?

Inulin is the only fiber that I use to rebalance or re-arrange bacterial overgrowth. I do not use or recommend the use of any other fibers, probiotics, vitamins, minerals, herbs, or enzymes for bacterial overgrowth for my patients. It is also not necessary to use supplements to reverse leaky gut as it will spontaneously repair itself within a few weeks of starting inulin (or treating with rifaximin)

Is testing for bacterial overgrowth, propionic acid, or types of bacteria in stools useful?

No. Although intriguing, medical science is nowhere close to understanding either how to do these tests accurately, nor do we understand the results in such a way that we could use the results to improve the treatment response in the child.

Warning:

My patients do not take probiotics during or after the use of inulin. The reason is that once the gut bacteria is rebalanced and the birds and the fish have shifted back to their respective environments, the last thing I want them to do is to introduce a foreign bacteria (like lizards) for their birds to have to deal with. There is growing evidence that the indiscriminate application of probiotics may worsen the overall blend of intestinal bacteria.

Preferred Method to Balance Gut Bacteria in Older Children and Adults:

Non-Absorbable Antibiotic
Rifaximin 550 mg twice daily for 10 days.

As children age, inulin is less and less effective at controlling the balance of intestinal bacteria. By the age of twenty, I have never witnessed the inulin being effective enough to assist in brain recovery.

If the child is between the ages of eight and fourteen, I may start with either inulin or rifaximin but if the child is fifteen or older, I recommend starting with rifaximin because of the low likelihood that inulin will be effective.

As children age, the inulin becomes less and less effective at controlling bacterial overgrowth. I believe this is due to the natural maturation of the intestinal bacteria as children mature into adulthood. We are not just trying to suppress "gut bacteria" as a singular entity, we are needing to suppress and balance over a thousand distinct species within the large intestine, all of which have their own unique characteristics.

The species of bacteria that tend to overgrow in the small intestine of a younger child (let us call them species A) may just tend to be more sensitive to the prebiotic effects of inulin. As a result, inulin is more effective in smaller children.

As the child's intestinal bacteria naturally mature with age, species that are less sensitive to the effects of inulin (let's call these species B) might be more likely to cause overgrowth and make inulin seem to lose its effectiveness in balancing the intestinal bacteria.

If inulin fiber loses its effectiveness over time, or the side effects (hyperactivity, anxiety, aggression) are intolerable, I recommend the use of rifaximin (brand name of Xifaxan® in the U.S.) 550 mg two times daily for 10 days to reduce the excessive colonic bacteria from the small intestine in my patients.

Safety Features of Rifaximin
- Not Absorbed into Bloodstream
- Side Effects are Very Uncommon
- Does No Damage to Intestinal Microbiome
- Bacteria Cannot Become Resistant to Rifaximin

Rifaximin will removal the abnormal presence of any colonic bacteria (species A as well as species B) that have overgrown within the small intestine yet does not harm the remaining colonic bacteria.

This is a prescription drug that must be prescribed and supervised by a physician. This pharmaceutical treatment may need to be periodically repeated as relapses of bacterial overgrowth can occur frequently.

Principles of Recovery

It is important to understand that treatment with inulin or rifaximin alone will not repair a child's brain and reversal of overgrowth will not control the primed M1-microglia and recovery will be limited. Aside from contributing an unhealthy amount of inflammatory stress within the brain, bacterial overgrowth also triggers the formation of primed M1-microglia that inhibit neuronal pruning, migration, and repair.

Supplementation with fish oil and olive oil and possibly the use of vagus nerve stimulation (VNS) may all be required to regulate inflammation and overcome the negative effects of the primed M1-microglia.

It is also important to mention that FMT (fecal microbiota therapy) has no direct effect bacterial overgrowth of the small intestine nor on the primed M1-microglia. As such, FMT will predictably have minimal effect on the restoration of neuronal pruning, neuronal migration, and cellular repair. I do not recommend FMT to my pediatric patients.

The key pathophysiological features of autism involve both brain inflammation and intestinal overgrowth and consistent effort is required to control both over the long term. The power of the protocol is in its collective impact on the reduction of inflammation within the brain.

Other than increasing the fish oil and olive oil doses as the child ages, altering or reducing the doses of individual components of the protocol often leads to confusion and may even reduce the protocol's effectiveness if mistakes are made.

Assessing Effectiveness

After completing the 10-day course of rifaximin and starting the fish oil and olive oil, parents will ask how they determine whether the doses are correct for their child. There are two things I look for when assessing the effectiveness of treatment.

First, the reversal of bacterial overgrowth with one course (10 days) of rifaximin will lead to a drop in propionic acid and often the awakening period. This is a period where the child becomes more aware, has more eye contact, more alertness, more engagement, but possibly may have more stimming or insomnia.

As I have stated before, the older the child, the less likely the parent will notice an awakening. This might be because the bacteria responsible for overgrowth in older children tend not to produce excessive propionic acid, or those species which do produce propionic acid have already been suppressed with dietary restrictions.

Secondly, if the intestinal bacteria blend has been rebalanced and the proper amounts of fish oil and olive oil are being given, there should be a noticeable increase in the rate of neurological development within the next few months.

If there is no significant improvement after 2-3 months, then I assume the intestinal bacteria are rapidly relapsing and more frequent dosing of rifaximin is needed.

Monitoring

Bacterial overgrowth of the small intestine is only sometimes detectable with a quantitative bacterial culture or PCR analysis of fluid aspiration from the small intestine, or by the abnormal metabolism of sugars with a hydrogen and/or methane breath test. Treatment with rifaximin often results in the reversal of the findings on these tests.

From a practical standpoint, these tests are not useful and I do not recommend they be performed on my patients. Quantitative culture and PCR analysis require a complicated endoscopy procedure each time a sample might be needed. The breath test has so many variables affecting its accuracy that the results are often more of a source of confusion rather than a source of clarity.

I quit using the breath test a long time ago with my patients because some would improve after rifaximin despite having an initial breath test that was negative for bacterial overgrowth.

Instead of these tests, I make very precise notes about the clinical improvements of intestinal, psychiatric, musculoskeletal, and neurological improvements my patients experience within the first month after treatment with inulin or rifaximin. This collective set of symptoms is what I referred to as the SIBO fingerprint.

I then use these changes in symptoms to check for bacterial overgrowth relapses because a relapse will often result in the return of many of the same symptoms that resolved originally on inulin or rifaximin.

Unfortunately, many children are often unable to communicate clearly enough to help us decode what they may be experiencing. And it is too often difficult for the parents to gauge any immediate changes by observation and the SIBO fingerprint approach becomes less useful.

Because of this challenge I use deductive reasoning to help me decide if the intestine's bacteria have been successfully balanced. I have learned that if inulin or rifaximin have been successful, noticeable developmental gains will become apparent within four to eight weeks.

If this does not occur especially by the third month, I then can reasonably conclude the inulin has failed or the child has rapidly relapsed after finishing the rifaximin.

. . .

Pointers and FAQ's:

Follow-up use of inulin after rifaximin is sometimes used if intestinal symptoms such as diarrhea, post-meal stool urgency, or food intolerance are still present. If inulin does not make any significant difference in these situations, I stop using it in my patients.

Rifaximin is a prescription medication and it should only be administered and supervised by a physician.

I never add probiotics to my patient's treatment program after rebalancing intestinal overgrowth with rifaximin because the addition of probiotics can easily make things worse for the patient, even if the probiotic seemed to help prior to the use of rifaximin. I have seen the addition of foreign strains of bacteria (probiotics) increase patients' inflammation, intestinal distress, depression, and other psychological symptoms.

Side Effects of Rifaximin

- Gas
- Headache
- Nausea
- Abdominal Cramps
- Persistent Diarrhea
- Blood or Mucus in Your Stool
- A Strong Desire to Have Bowel Movement
- Ineffective, Painful, Straining of Stool or Urine

Except when using inulin for continued diarrhea, etc., the continued use of prebiotic fibers such as inulin, probiotics, or digestive enzymes after taking rifaximin is strongly discouraged because they may cause a worsening of symptoms after intestinal bacterial re-balancing is achieved.

Step Two: Reduction of Brain Inflammation

In the earlier chapter, I explained how cytokines from bacterial translocation are reduced with the rebalancing of intestinal bacteria in Step 1 with inulin or rifaximin. In this section, I will explain the components involved in further reducing inflammation with The Nemechek Protocol®.

In addition to the release of pro-inflammatory cytokines from bacterial overgrowth, there are four additional sources of inflammation that need to be addressed each in their own unique manner.

Lowering Four Additional Sources of Inflammation

- Shift M1-Microglia towards the Anti-Inflammatory M2-Microglia Phenotype
- Balance Omega-6 and Omega-3 Fatty Acids
- Reduction of Dietary Linoleic, Arachidonic, and Palmitic Acids
- Improving Vagus Nerve Function

Shifting M1-Microglia to the Anti-Inflammatory M2-Phenotype

Increasing the intake of omega-3 fatty acids is a critical step and must be performed to shift inflammatory primed M1-microglia to the anti-inflammatory M2-microglial phenotype.

The M1 to M2 shift maximizes the brain's natural ability to restore proper neurological development by re-initiating synaptic pruning, neuronal migration, and neuronal repair as well as ensure maximum recovery.

The human body requires a blend of omega-3 fatty acids which are the core nutrients that earlier generations obtained in their everyday foods but are now commonly lacking in the modern food supply.

There are three types of omega-3 and each has distinct functions: DHA, EPA, and ALA. DHA is docosahexaenoic acid, EPA is eicosapentaenoic acid, and ALA is alpha-linolenic acid.

All three types of omega-3 are important but for this part of The Nemechek Protocol® we focus on the DHA component in particular for its ability to aid in the repair of brain damage from inflammation and injury. DHA is the only omega-3 fatty acid that substantially penetrates the brain and is found in variable amounts in fish oil.

Patients must supplement with DHA in order to shift their primed M1-microglia cells back into the M2-microglia type that allows proper brain development and recovery from cumulative brain injury. There are no substitutes for the DHA omega-3 fatty acid supplementation.

The amounts of daily DHA that I use with my patients may be taken all at once or they may be taken in divided doses throughout the day. They can also be taken with or without food. Although important in its own right, the specific amount of accompanying EPA that is paired with the DHA component in fish oil is less critical. This might be because EPA does not readily penetrate the central nervous system.

At this time, I recommend high concentration DHA fish oil pills or liquids that are available from NOW® Foods or Nordic Naturals® and these specific brands are listed in the appendix. These are the brands I preferentially use to help my patients recover from a wide variety of neurological impairment and injury. Cod liver oil also works well when supplementing omega-3 fatty acids, and it is dosed in the same manner as regular fish oil.

I recommend against using the new high DHA concentration formulations that contain little to no EPA. Although little EPA enters the central nervous system, its presence in the fish oil blends I recommend is important for the proper function of cells outside of the central nervous system.

Balancing Omega-3 and Omega-6 Fatty Acids

This chart contains the dosage of Nordic Naturals Ultimate Omega fish oil I commonly recommend for my patients based on their age.

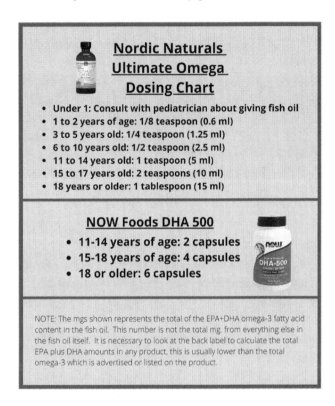

Nordic Naturals
Ultimate Omega
Dosing Chart

- Under 1: Consult with pediatrician about giving fish oil
- 1 to 2 years of age: 1/8 teaspoon (0.6 ml)
- 3 to 5 years old: 1/4 teaspoon (1.25 ml)
- 6 to 10 years old: 1/2 teaspoon (2.5 ml)
- 11 to 14 years old: 1 teaspoon (5 ml)
- 15 to 17 years old: 2 teaspoons (10 ml)
- 18 years or older: 1 tablespoon (15 ml)

NOW Foods DHA 500

- 11-14 years of age: 2 capsules
- 15-18 years of age: 4 capsules
- 18 or older: 6 capsules

NOTE: The mgs shown represents the total of the EPA+DHA omega-3 fatty acid content in the fish oil. This number is not the total mg. from everything else in the fish oil itself. It is necessary to look at the back label to calculate the total EPA plus DHA amounts in any product, this is usually lower than the total omega-3 which is advertised or listed on the product.

Alternatively, teens and adults who can swallow fish oil capsules can use DHA-500 from NOW Foods, Inc.

Pointers:

Does fish oil cause intestinal distress?

Sometimes my patients may experience loose stools that can occur when first starting their fish oil. This is often due to their intestinal tract being irritated from bacterial overgrowth or not being able to absorb the sudden increase of oil being ingested.

If loose stools occur, I will have my patients stop their fish oil for two to three weeks until the rebalancing of their intestinal bacteria with inulin or rifaximin gives their intestinal tract a chance to repair itself. Then after a few weeks, my patients can restart their fish oil at a 1/4 of the full dose.

They may slowly increase the dosage by adding another ¼ dose every week or so until they reach the full dose. The reason for this is that by slowly increasing the amount of fish oil, we essentially train the intestinal tract to increase its ability to absorb the fatty acid molecules in the oil.

Do I ever add vitamins or products in addition to fish oil in my patients?

No. The addition of supplements such as glutamine, digestive enzymes, biofilm agents, or anti-fungal medications are not necessary for intestinal bacteria recovery from bacterial overgrowth or the absorption of fish oil.

An exception to this rule is the supplementation of iron or a particular vitamin by a medical physician in response to documented low levels.

Do I ever use fermented fish oil with my patients?

No. I do not recommend fermented fish oil.

Do I ever use krill oil with my patients?

No. Krill oil is a different molecule than the fish oil molecule. Our ancestors evolved on the shorter molecule that is found in fish oil, not on the longer molecule found in krill oil. I use the exact same molecules and core nutrients that kept our ancestor's brains strong and resilient. These happen to be much less expensive in the doses we require than commonly are available from krill oil.

Is there a vegetarian option if your patients are allergic to fish or do not want to ingest a fish byproduct?

Maybe. There is algae-derived DHA which might be beneficial but I have never seen any of my patients on algae-derived DHA significantly improve.

Autonomic improvement and recovery were believed to be medically impossible until I developed The Nemechek Protocol® and have only been realized with marine-based DHA. The lack of EPA in algae derived DHA might be a reason for it not seeming to work.

Can another form of omega-3 (EPA or ALA) substitute for the DHA from fish?

No. Other forms of non-marine omega-3 fatty acids, such as flax oil (ALA), do not readily penetrate the central nervous system and do not have the same impact on inflammation or microglia function as DHA.

The Additional of Alpha-Linoleic Acid (ALA)

The third component of omega-3 is ALA, (alpha-linolenic acid), which is plant-based omega-3. There is some research that suggests ALA may help DHA penetrate into the brain.

I recommend patients eighteen years or older on The Nemechek Protocol® take some form of daily supplementation of omega-3 ALA either from nuts (dry-roasted), flax, or ground chia seeds, as long as they are not allergic to any of those items.

If my patients chose to consume nuts as part of The Nemechek Protocol®, I instruct them to eat a minimum of ¼ cup of nuts per day. All tree nuts have adequate supplies of ALA and these include almonds, pecans, pistachios, cashews, and walnuts. Dry or roasted peanuts (which are legumes and are not tree nuts) are an acceptable ALA source as well.

If my patient decides to consume ALA by ground flaxseed or chia seeds, they will supplement with 1/2 to 1 tablespoon per day. If they are consuming flax oil in liquid or soft gel form, the amount is between 500 to 1,000 mg once daily.

Reducing the Dietary Intake of Omega-6 Fatty Acids

Reducing pro-inflammatory cytokines with The Nemechek Protocol® also requires a decrease in the patient's dietary intake of high concentration omega-6 fatty acid cooking oils.

This is done both by no longer cooking with them (vegetable oils, margarine, shortening), and by eliminating foods that contain high linoleic acid oils as primary ingredients.

I instruct my patients to avoid consuming food products that contain omega-6 fatty acids. Try to avoid consuming these when possible. If you get a little bit in your diet here and there, the daily consumption of olive oil will protect you.

Prohibited Oils:
- Soy (Soybean) Oil
- Sunflower Oil
- Corn Oil
- Safflower Oil
- Cottonseed Oil
- Grapeseed Oil
- Peanut Oil
- Margarine
- Shortening

Foods containing soy milk or soy protein or lethicin are allowed if they do not also list any of the prohibited oils on the label. In these first stages of The Nemechek Protocol®, the reduction of omega-6 oils from foods is often the most demanding thing for my patients to do.

If the food product contains any of those prohibited oils listed above, I recommend reducing their intake as much as is practical or replacing them with a different brand that contains an acceptable oil. There are a few oils that have a healthier balance of omega-6 to omega-3 fatty acid ratio and are preferred for general cooking.

Acceptable Oils

- Canola Oil
- Coconut Oil
- Avocado Oil
- Palm Kernel Oil

Once my patients start reading labels for omega-6 oils, it becomes clear to them the extent that these oils now appear in foods that they eat every day such as salad dressings and bread. Omega-6 oils can be found in foods that we may otherwise consider to be clean, organic, and healthy. They even appear as ingredients in pet foods.

Pointer:

Memorize the acceptable oils, it is easier than trying to memorize the longer list of prohibited oils. Canola is increasingly being used in store-bought foods because of its healthier profile. One of my mottos is, "My patients *can* have *can*ola oil."

Some products will say that they contain either a prohibited or an acceptable oil (e.g. "may contain soybean oil or canola oil"). The consumer is left to wonder which oil is being used in the product. I personally err on the side of caution and try to avoid products whose ingredients are not clear to me.

Prevention of Brain and Systemic Inflammation from Dietary Linoleic, Arachidonic and Palmitic Acids

While on The Nemechek Protocol®, I recommend patients try to avoid omega-6 fatty acids in cooking oils and foods but also to protect themselves from omega-6 that they cannot control.

There are three specific omega-6 fatty acids that are common within the food supply and should be avoided if possible because excessive intake can contribute to excessive inflammation.

- **Linoleic acid** - commonly found in the unnatural vegetable oils added to the foods we purchased in the market.
- **Arachidonic acid** - found in elevated concentrations in dietary meats that are fed grains such as soybeans or corn.
- **Palmitic acid** - found in high quantities in processed foods as well as grain-fed foods.

Patients find these hard to control because they may not be able to see them on an ingredient label They may not know what was fed to the meat or fish they eat, or they do not know what type of cooking oils are being used by a restaurant.

Fortunately, the omega-9 fatty acid oleic acid is capable of blocking the inflammatory toxicity of these omega-6 fatty acids and high quantities of oleic acid is present in authentic extra virgin olive oil.

The daily consumption of omega-9 rich olive oil is an essential step in protecting the body from excessive omega-6 fatty acid toxicity.

Daily Supplementation with Olive Oil

In addition to decreasing the consumption of high concentration omega-6 fatty acid cooking oils and foods, I ask my patients to increase their daily consumption of extra virgin olive oil (EVOO). EVOO contains approximately 70% oleic acid, and oleic acid is capable of reducing the underlying inflammation resulting from excessive dietary intakes of linoleic, arachidonic and palmitic acid.

Several studies show that adults benefit from the daily consumption of two or more tablespoons (30 ml or more) of extra virgin olive oil daily. Increasing your intake of EVOO can be done by topping foods with olive oil in the traditional manner or by simply drinking it straight as if it were a medicine.

Heating olive oil while cooking does not damage the oleic acid molecule nor lower the amount contained within the oil.

For children less than three years old, I believe that using EVOO when cooking foods should be an adequate amount. Starting at age three, I recommend supplementing the diet by adding EVOO to food or directly consuming it. These are the following guidelines:

- If under 2 years of age, cooking food daily in EVOO should be adequate
- If between 2 to 4 years old, give ¼-½ of a teaspoon (1.25-2.5 ml) of EVOO daily
- If between 4 to 8 years old, give 1 teaspoon (5 ml) of EVOO daily
- If between 9 to 12 years old, give 2 teaspoons (10 ml) of EVOO daily
- If between 13 to 17 years old, give 1 tablespoon (15 ml) of EVOO daily
- If 18 years or older, give 2 tablespoons (30 ml) of EVOO daily

Pointer:

EVOO may be mixed into a variety of liquids or taken by spoon. Some of my older patients cut the taste with a drop of balsamic or lemon juice.

EVOO is not well regulated in the U.S. and the risk of buying oils that are not actually extra virgin or are tainted with other oils is a great concern for my patients. Some olive oils may be diluted with a high percentage of soy oil or other vegetable oils, the very things we are trying to avoid.

Because of the considerable risk of buying fraudulent imported olive oils, patients on The Nemechek Protocol® are recommended to use extra virgin olive oils certified by the California Olive Oil Council (COOC; www.cooc.com for more information).

COOC-certification is the only certification process in the U.S. that requires laboratory testing of olive oil to prove the purity and quality of the oil. You can find approved COOC-certified producers and their certification of EVOO off the COOC.com website, and have the products shipped to your home to avoid deterioration of a product not properly stored in a grocery stores warehouse.

Improving Vagus Nerve Function

The vagus nerve is the tenth cranial nerve and carries information from the parasympathetic branch of the autonomic nervous system. Neurological signals on the vagus nerve travel both upwards into the brain and downwards to all the organs in the body. Signals traveling upwards are capable of inducing neuroplasticity while signals traveling downward improve organ function and help suppress abnormal levels of inflammation.

Vagus nerve stimulation (VNS) is a treatment that involves extremely low electrical impulses to the vagus nerve. Vagus nerve stimulators have been implanted in patients in the U.S. since the late 1990s, but it is also possible to stimulate the nerve externally.

I use a portable vagus nerve stimulator as part of The Nemechek Protocol® that many of my autistic and non-autistic patients use at home.

VNS results in the suppression of inflammation as well as increased neuroplasticity especially when paired with a cognitive (speech, reading, mathematics training), sensory (integration therapy), or motor (physical therapy or gait training) activity.

The use of transcutaneous (across the skin) Vagus nerve stimulation (tVNS) for 5 minutes per day is an extremely powerful and effective tool for the suppression of inflammation as well as for the induction of neuroplasticity. The suppression of inflammation within the brain improves the brain repair and neuronal pruning abilities of microglia.

I may add tVNS to a child's treatment at a later stage in The Nemechek Protocol® if their recovery is incomplete or unusually slow. Once recovery has begun, tVNS treatment may help expand the breadth of a child's recovery.

While all children are treated with identical stimulation parameters, my adult patients use tVNS with a variety different settings based on several factors that I take under consideration as their doctor.

Transcutaneous VNS can cause harm if the stimulation settings are incorrect. I am a leading expert in the clinical application of tVNS and many of my patients travel to my office in Arizona to be prescribed a portable transcutaneous vagus nerve stimulator they can use at home. The are other neuromodulators such as Gamma-Core, and wellness products like the Vitality Smartcable, that are comparable devices.

I do not prescribe or perform any other non-electrical methods of vagus stimulation because other methods are less effective at keeping the healthy shift in microglia function.

Pointer:

The need for tVNS increases with the severity of developmental impairment as well as the age of the patient. By the early teen years, it seems most children with autism or developmental disorders may require tVNS in order to obtain a full, broad level of neurological recovery.

Warning:

I also strongly recommend against any tVNS do-it-yourself approach using other devices such as TENS units because of the potential harm that may occur if not set or used correctly. The vagus nerve may be permanently damaged is stimulation is done incorrectly.

18

THE HISTORY OF BALANCING THE INTESTINAL TRACT

Although bacterial overgrowth of the small intestine (SIBO) has garnered growing attention in recent years, intestinal bacterial overgrowth is a medical problem that was discovered approximately sixty years ago.

While The Nemechek Protocol® is a relatively new approach to reversing the toxic and inflammatory effects of bacterial overgrowth to treat autism, the techniques and medications described in this book were developed over many decades in the treatment of adults with other forms of bacterial overgrowth.

The purpose of this chapter is to highlight the parallels between existing and widely accepted techniques for the treatment of bacterial overgrowth and the use of rifaximin in The Nemechek Protocol® for the same purpose.

Bacterial Overgrowth has a Long History

Some of the first medical studies involved the treatment of bacterial overgrowth in patients with advanced cirrhosis of the liver (hepatic encephalopathy) in the 1960s and later with overgrowth of a particular bacterium, *Clostridium difficle* (*C. difficle* enterocolitis and pseudomembranous colitis) in the late 1970s.

Since untreated hepatic encephalopathy and *C. difficle* enterocolitis are potentially deadly, a great deal of medical research exists on how to medically manage bacterial overgrowth associated with these conditions.

The use of antibiotics (vancomycin and metronidazole) for the management of *C. difficle* enterocolitis will be discussed in parallel with the use of rifaximin to control overgrowth in children with autism, developmental delay, and cumulative brain injury, to show that this approach to bacterial overgrowth has been widely accepted by the medical community for years.

Clostridium difficle Enterocolitis

Clostridium difficle (*C. difficle*) is a bacteria that can be found living harmlessly within the lower portion of the intestinal tract (i.e., large intestine or colon) along with a thousand or so of other bacterial species.

When restricted to the lower intestine in small numbers, *C. difficle* is harmless because its growth is regulated by the counterbalancing effects of the other bacteria also living within the colon.

When a bacterial overgrowth of the small intestine occurs, the overgrowth is generally from a single species of bacteria that normally lives within the colon but now is growing in much greater numbers within the small intestine.

Normally the small intestine has very few bacteria within it and as such, they are unable to restrict the growth of the intruding bacterium from the colon.

The intruding colonic bacterium will grow unregulated until 10,000-100,000 times the normal bacteria are living within the small intestine. Excessive bacteria within the small intestine will damage tissue leading to nutrient malabsorption as well as inflammation from bacterial translocation (i.e., leaky gut). The overgrowth can also disrupt the nervous, hormone, and immune systems throughout the body.

These excessive bacteria have the potential to begin producing abnormal types or amounts of chemicals that are programmed into their genetic material. As the concentrations of these chemicals increase, they end up circulating in the bloodstream and produce negative effects on the body. In the specific case of *C. difficle*, the chemicals produced from the overgrowth are called Toxin A and Toxin B.

When released, Toxin A and Toxin B trigger a severe inflammatory reaction that damages the small intestine and colon resulting in fever, fatigue, abdominal pain, and severe diarrhea and if left untreated will eventually lead to shock and death.

Clostridium enterocolitis is simple bacterial overgrowth with a particular strain of deadly bacteria called *Clostridium difficle*.

Similarities Managing SIBO with The Nemechek Protocol® and Enterocolitis

The escalating frequency of rifaximin use I recommend with my protocol is similar to the escalating frequency of courses of antibiotics used in *C. difficle* enterocolitis.

In patients suffering from *C. difficle* enterocolitis, antibiotics are used to help control *C. difficle*. The initial approach is to treat with a single ten-to-fourteen-day course of antibiotic.

For many patients, their diarrhea, fever, and abdominal pain will resolve and never return. Similarly, an initial approach of The Nemechek Protocol® is to use a single course of rifaximin.

In *C. difficle* enterocolitis, some patients will quickly relapse after discontinuing the antibiotics. The relapses then require physicians to use repeated courses of antibiotics to control *C. difficle*. Eventually, the relapses of *C. difficle* overgrowth in most patients will cease after a few to several cycles of antibiotics.

Single Course of Antibiotic -> Several Cycles of Antibiotics

Adults with SIBO also experience relapses of bacterial overgrowth and may also require repeated courses of rifaximin. I have my adult patients repeat their 10-day course of rifaximin whenever their symptoms return (heartburn, diarrhea, joint or abdominal pain, etc.) for more than 10-14 days. Similar to *C. difficle* enterocolitis, patients relapsing with SIBO will eventually stop relapsing after a few to several cycles of rifaximin.

My approach to treating children with relapsing bacterial overgrowth is similar but different in one respect. Children are often unable to readily communicate the internal symptoms that improved with a course of rifaximin and likewise, cannot communicate when the symptoms have returned.

Unfortunately, they may relapse before any outward improvements can be observed by their parents. Therefore, the determination of when to repeat rifaximin as determined by the parents proved ineffective.

Since the inflammatory stress of intestinal bacterial overgrowth prevents any further neurological recovery, I deduced that the children who did not show increased recovery after a single course of rifaximin were relapsing very quickly. I devised a system of monthly cycles of rifaximin to maintain the balance of bacteria within their intestinal tract.

But even cycles of antibiotics might not be enough to eventually stop the relapses common with *C. difficle* enterocolitis or bacterial overgrowth in children and adults.

In the case of rapidly recurring enterocolitis, infectious disease specialists might prescribe a continuous round of antibiotics for one to several months. The Nemechek Protocol® takes the same approach with children.

Cycles of Antibiotics -> Continuous Course of Antibiotics

If a child is not demonstrating substantial neurological recovery with *monthly* cycles of rifaximin, they are experiencing a relapse of bacterial overgrowth often within a week after completing the rifaximin.

I first observed this with some extremely aggressive autistic patients I have worked with. Within a few days of starting rifaximin, the violent tendencies in some of these patients would greatly diminish but the aggression would return within a week after finishing the 10-day course of rifaximin.

The return of aggression after every cycle of rifaximin was consistent round after round. Once continuous rifaximin was begun, the aggression was consistently improved and within two to three months significant signs of neurological recovery began indicating to me that bacterial overgrowth was finally suppressed.

After twelve months of rifaximin therapy, most patients could be tapered back from monthly cycles to intermittent rifaximin or from continuous to monthly cycles of rifaximin then eventually to intermittent rifaximin.

Tapering Can Occur Often After 12 Months
Continuous Rifaximin -> Monthly Rifaximin -> Intermittent Rifaximin

In conjunction with the other aspects of The Nemechek Protocol®, a child's' recovery with more aggressive use of rifaximin has been exceptionally positive. Many parents are opting to maintain some sort of controlling rifaximin to avoid relapses and continue the exciting recovery path their child is experiencing.

FMT and C. Difficle Enterocolitis

There are patients with *C. difficle* enterocolitis that do not even respond to continuous antibiotics who will eventually deteriorate and die of septic shock. For decades treatment-resistant enterocolitis killed thousands of patients in the U.S. every year.

Within the last several years, a treatment referred to as fecal microbiota transplant (FMT) has been discovered to control treatment-resistant enterocolitis. FMT entails increasing the diversity of bacteria within the patient's intestinal track with a specimen of fecal stool from a healthy donor.

Continuous Course of Antibiotics -> Fecal Microbiota Transplant

By recolonizing the bacteria in this manner, patients near-death from treatment-resistant *C. difficle* quite miraculously recover within only a few days. The patients who eventually require FMT often have very low levels of bacterial biodiversity within their intestinal tract.

The effectiveness of FMT in this scenario underscores the importance of how the other intestinal bacteria are a critical component in the re-establishment of bacterial balance within the intestinal tract.

Rifaximin and other antibiotics do not force bacterial intestinal balance to occur, they shift the balance of bacteria back in the right direction, so the remaining bacteria are able to regulate the balance themselves.

Aside from a dramatic improvement in patients with treatment-resistant *C. difficle* enterocolitis, FMT has had relatively limited success in treating patients with inflammatory bowel disease, obesity, or diabetes.

In my experience, it is rare that a child does not respond to either inulin or rifaximin (cycling or continuous). Therefore, I am uncertain if there is any significant utility of FMT in children with autism, developmental delay, or cumulative brain injury.

In support of my skepticism, intestinal bacterial studies of children with autism do not detect low levels of biodiversity as found in adults with recurrent *C. difficle* enterocolitis. Furthermore, I have many children under my care who have been treated with FMT by other physicians with little to no significant success.

Applying Old Science to a New Scenario

As we have reviewed, the manner in which The Nemechek Protocol® recommends either a single course of rifaximin, cycles of rifaximin, and potentially even a continuous course of rifaximin to control disabling bacterial overgrowth in children parallels what has been done for decades in adults.

The focus of The Nemechek Protocol® is to safely induce neurological recovery in the children by controlling inflammation and bacterial overgrowth with techniques developed over decades for adults.

19

PANS, AND PANDAS, AND AUTISM

DIFFERENT FACES OF THE SAME DISORDER

The last few decades have seen an alarming increase in acquired neurological disorders among children. Children are increasingly developing conditions such as autism, developmental delay, sensory problems, emotional disorders, attention disorders (ADD/ADHD), post-concussion syndrome, tics, Tourette's syndrome, and PANS, and PANDAS. Acquired neurological conditions developed after birth and are view differently from congenital disorders that may have a genetic component or have occurred before birth.

Consequently, researchers are grappling to understand each of these conditions, but unfortunately, they often focus on individual disorders and not the bigger picture. There is little to no research on understanding why such a large variety of neurological conditions are increasingly affecting children over the same time frame.

<u>Commonly Acquired Neurological Conditions</u>
Tics
Autism
PANS/PANDAS
Attention Disorders
Emotional Disorders
Tourette's Syndrome
Developmental Disorders
Post-Concussion Syndrome

When assessing an individual who develops a variety of symptoms within a relatively narrow timeframe, a physician is trained not to view each problem or symptom separately but to look for a single cause that might be responsible for all their symptoms. Applying the same logic to the increase of the acquired neurological issues in children, I think small intestine bacterial overgrowth (SIBO) could be the single common factor contributing to all of these conditions.

SIBO is a condition in which bacteria that typically live within the colon are found in high concentrations within the small intestine. The small intestine typically has relatively few bacteria but SIBO results in bacterial counts ranging from 1,000 – 100,000 times the amount normally found. Besides contributing to some digestive issues such as diarrhea, reflux, and food intolerance, SIBO results in leakage of molecules of nutrients and bacteria into tissue layers surrounding the small intestine.

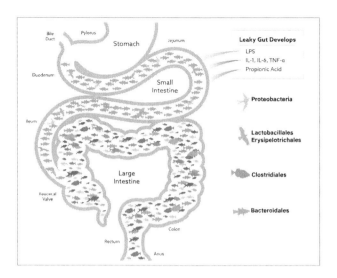

The small intestine wall disruption is referred to as bacterial translocation (i.e., leaky gut) since only bacteria cause this. Yeast (i.e., fungi, Candida), viruses, and protozoa (i.e., parasites) may grow in excess within the small intestine, but there is no evidence they contribute to the leaky gut problem.

I can explain SIBO's ability to trigger various neurological disorders in children through two factors, the age when bacterial overgrowth first occurs and whether or not the overgrowing bacteria can produce a behavior-altering substance such as propionic acid.

For normal neurological development in a child to occur, the brain's neuron mass is pruned from approximately 100 billion neurons down to 50 billion by the time the child is five years old. Inflammation from SIBO can prevent the pruning from occurring correctly. If SIBO occurs before five years of age, the child will have some developmental or sensory issue. If it occurs after five years of age, no developmental problems arise because the pruning is already complete.

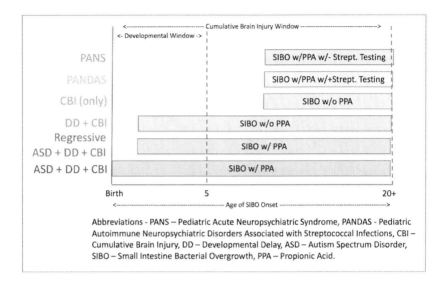

Abbreviations - PANS – Pediatric Acute Neuropsychiatric Syndrome, PANDAS - Pediatric Autoimmune Neuropsychiatric Disorders Associated with Streptococcal Infections, CBI – Cumulative Brain Injury, DD – Developmental Delay, ASD – Autism Spectrum Disorder, SIBO – Small Intestine Bacterial Overgrowth, PPA – Propionic Acid.

When SIBO is present, unresolved residual neurological damage remains after each injury. Over time, the unresolved injury from repeated traumas will build on top of each other, resulting in a cumulative brain injury or CBI phenomenon.

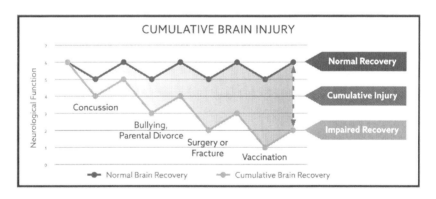

CBI's symptoms or behaviors include hyperactivity, anxiety, chronic depression, excessive aggression, poor focus, heartburn, reflux, and constipation.

Unlike the pruning process, cumulative brain injuries can occur throughout the entire life span. Therefore, whether or not the inflammation from SIBO occurs before or after age five, CBI increases with each additional injury.

SIBO Before 5 Years of Age

If SIBO occurs after the age of 5, a child can only develop cumulative brain injury. If SIBO occurs before the age of 5, the child will always experience CBI and developmental delay. Depending on the intensity of the inflammatory strain caused by SIBO, the developmental issue can be mild or severe.

Propionic acid (PPA) is found in high concentration in the tissues of children with advanced autism and has a sedating, and at times almost hallucinatory, effect on the children. The production of PPA is dependent on the specific colonic bacteria that is overgrown within the small intestine. Since not all colonic bacteria produce propionic acid, the excess production of PPA depends on whether or not the overgrowing species is capable of excreting it. If the overgrowing bacteria produce PPA, the child will have a decreased level of awareness, poor eye contact, and may engage in strange behaviors such as staring transfixed at spinning objects.

In a child younger than five years old with SIBO with a PPA-producing species of bacteria, that child will have developmental issues, cumulative brain injury symptoms, and behaviors uniquely associated with autism. If younger than the age of five when SIBO occurs with a bacteria that does not produce PPA, then the child will not have these unique autistic behaviors and will only be diagnosed with developmental delay and cumulative brain injury.

SIBO After 5 Years of Age

After the age of five, the occurrence of SIBO without PPA production will result in cumulative brain injury symptoms and no developmental issues. In the event the child is older than five years old, SIBO occurs with PPA-producing bacteria, they will manifest in conditions commonly referred to as PANS (pediatric acute-onset neuropsychiatric syndrome) or PANDAS (pediatric autoimmune neuropsychiatric disorder associated with streptococcal infections).

The symptoms commonly felt to be associated with PANS and PANDAS both consist of high levels of anxiety, often resulting in obsessive-compulsive behaviors (i.e., OCD) and a variety of other neurological and psychiatric symptoms. The main difference between the two is that PANS has a rapid onset, often within 24-48 hours. In contrast, PANDAS does not develop rapidly and is associated with the colonization of streptococcal bacteria in the pharynx (i.e., a positive strep throat swab). Both PANS and PANDAS can

220

mysteriously disappear as quickly as they appear and then reappear months or years later.

I believe both PANS and PANDAS are simply the occurrence of SIBO with PPA-producing bacteria and are not separate medical conditions. In animal studies, SIBO increases anxiety-like behavior, and I have witnessed this same effect in my private practice. A subset of my adult patients will also experience high levels of anxiety after SIBO develops. The anxiety can rapidly resolve after treatment of SIBO with rifaximin (Xifaxan®). Many of these adults had their anxiety initially escalate very rapidly after an infection, a course of antibiotics, surgery, or a brain injury, all of which are well-known triggers of SIBO.

The confusion with PANS and PANDAS is that the spontaneous resolution of these conditions after a course of antibiotics lies in commonly used antibiotics such as amoxicillin or trimethoprim/sulfamethoxazole have a 20-30% chance of reversing SIBO. Thus, their use can sometimes lead to rapid improvement of symptoms and even result in complete remission of symptoms sometimes.

Suppose a physician managing child with PANS or PANDAS is not tracking every single course of antibiotics that any other physicians might have prescribed the same patient for a routine middle ear or dental infection. The common antibiotics used in these instances can reverse SIBO and trigger an improvement in the patient's PANS or PANDA symptoms. The physician commonly misses the real reason for the child's improving symptoms and considers their progress as "spontaneous" or a consequence of some other treatment (vitamins, homeopathy, heavy metal therapy, etc.).

Positive Strep Tests Don't Always Mean What You Think

Also, the diagnosis of PANDAS requires the presence of a positive streptococcal throat test or culture in children. Approximately 10% of all children within the U.S. are carriers of harmless strains of streptococcus, test positive with rapid strept tests or throat cultures, and do not have any symptoms. Infectious disease specialists advise against treating these children with antibiotics because they are often incapable of clearing the streptococcus and do not benefit their health.

Because of the high carrier rate, 10% of any group of children with any common disorder will carry streptococcus. Because of this, streptococcus can mistakenly be linked to almost any disease process using this logic. What further leads physicians down this path of mistaken therapy is that prolonged courses of antibiotics they treat children with can partially suppress SIBO and reduce PPA production, resulting in some improvement in the child's symptoms.

The faulty logic of "giving antibiotics for streptococcus bacteria leads to improvement; therefore, the problem is caused by streptococcus" is understandable but incorrect. Treating the same child with rifaximin has a better and longer-lasting positive response. And since rifaximin does not enter the bloodstream, the positive impact from rifaximin cannot be because it cleared the throat's streptococcus infection.

Autoimmune Versus Autoinflammatory

While I agree that children diagnosed with PANS or PANDAS have excess inflammation within their brains, I disagree that this is an autoimmune process; the children suffer from an autoinflammatory process. Inflammation from an autoimmune process targets specific types of tissue in the body. For example, rheumatoid arthritis is an autoimmune disorder in which inflammation is primary located in just a few particular joints of the hands. Think of autoimmunity as a sharpshooter who can hit the center of a bullseye when shooting a bullet without damaging other bodily systems.

Autoinflammation is the release of inflammatory chemicals into the bloodstream, and these chemicals have wide-ranging adverse effects on the tissue of the body. In the case of the hands, almost all the joints of the hand would hurt, and not just a specific few joints as seen in rheumatoid arthritis. Instead of a sharpshooter, think of autoinflammation as a shotgun that cannot hit just the center of the target but instead scatters its effect across a much larger area.

When SIBO is present, the leakage through the small intestine walls can activate up to 80% of all white blood cells. These cells, in turn, release inflammatory chemicals called cytokines into the bloodstream and potentially harm any cell from head to toe.

Besides, reversal of SIBO with rifaximin causes a rapid reduction in autoinflammation and PPA levels and results in the sudden improvement of my patients mistakenly diagnosed with PANS and PANDAS. Historically, the treatment of most autoimmune disorders results in a slow reversal of a patient's symptoms.

The Effectiveness of the Nemechek Protocol®

I have assisted in the care of almost 700 children with autism, developmental delay, sensory issues, and cumulative brain injury, many of which had been previously diagnosed and treated for PANS or PANDAS. The Nemechek Protocol® is solely focused on reducing inflammation and most notably through the reversal of SIBO using either the prebiotic fiber inulin or the non-absorbable antibiotic rifaximin.

My protocol allows more than 90% of the children under my care to maintain a rate of neurological recovery that parents, teachers, and therapists find unequaled. My protocol's true power and success lie within the human body's natural ability to neurologically recover if the body is maintained in a healthy, non-inflammatory state.

PART VI

THINKING ABOUT THE FUTURE

20

POTENTIAL OPPORTUNITIES FOR PREVENTION

Now that I have discovered a process that can reverse or improve key features in existing autism and many other childhood disorders, I naturally consider whether this same process may be used in a potentially preventive manner. If I can make a change in the children of today, what about making a change in the children of tomorrow?

The prevention of inflammation and bacterial overgrowth might be key targets in the prevention of many childhood developmental disorders. In the case of autism, the first challenge is whether we can prevent the excessive production of propionic acid from bacterial overgrowth as it is the unique pathological feature that delineates autism from most other disorders.

If we can keep a child's intestinal bacteria balanced without over-growth in the small intestine and excessive production of propionic acid, autism, developmental delay and cumulative brain injury in most children would likely not occur.

In this chapter, I have included the recommendations I discuss with my patients that address potential methods to limit or reduce the risk of a child from developing clinically harmful overgrowth of intestinal bacterial.

None of my prevention suggestions in this chapter are "proven" in the sense that human clinical trials have been performed. My theories come from my experiences and observations after treating adults of all ages, children with autism and developmental disorders, and women before and after pregnancy with The Nemechek Protocol®.

I have been able to reverse or greatly improve the bacterial overgrowth in mothers of child-bearing age and children of all ages. There is reasonable potential that the same methods that prevent bacterial overgrowth might also prevent or limit the occurrence of autism, developmental delay and cumulative brain injury since they are commonly the consequence of bacterial overgrowth.

Any readers of this book who are learning about the treatment modalities and suggestions that I give to my patients must fully discuss any and all of these potential treatment modalities and suggestions with their healthcare providers before initiating them at any time prior conceiving, during pregnancy, or after delivery.

Considerations Before Pregnancy

Women considering pregnancy need to be aware that pro-inflammatory cytokines (IL-1, IL-6, TNF-alpha) that are produced within their body can cross the placenta and cause potential harm to their unborn child.

Pro-inflammatory cytokines can disrupt normal brain development as well as activating genes in their child while still within the womb and after birth. After birth, they may even be capable of causing new mutations within the child's DNA. These cytokines are also associated with increased pregnancy complications such as miscarriage and eclampsia.

I recommend my female patients who are considering becoming pregnant to work towards normalizing their body's inflammatory status many months before planning to conceive. The Nemechek Protocol® for Autonomic Recovery (for adults) is designed to specifically reduce a person's excessive levels of pro-inflammatory cytokines to improve or restore autonomic nervous system dysfunction.

Waiting until a woman becomes pregnant before starting the process of general inflammation reduction is not a good strategy because it may take three or more months to achieve a lower or normal state of inflammatory cytokines and both rifaximin and vagus nerve stimulation are prohibited from use during pregnancy and inulin supplementation is less effective in adults..

The higher dietary consumptions of olive oil and fish as part of the Mediterranean diet are associated with favorable neurobehavioral outcomes in early childhood. There is no reason to believe the olive oil and fish oil recommended with The Nemechek Protocol® would not offer the same benefits.

The rifaximin medication I prescribe to my adult patients to reverse intestinal bacterial overgrowth is not a treatment option during pregnancy as it is not approved for use during pregnancy or breastfeeding.

The reduction of overall inflammation prior to pregnancy may improve fertility rates and limit complications such as pre-eclampsia and miscarriage during pregnancy. Supplementing with fish oil and olive oil can also increase the mother's neurological resilience against the intense physical and psychological stressors that accompany delivery.

Ensuring a woman does not have significant bacterial overgrowth and supplementing their diet with the correct balance of omega-3 and omega-6 fatty acids via The Nemechek Protocol® will go a long way towards maximizing their chances for a healthy and uncomplicated pregnancy.

Considerations During Pregnancy

Inflammation can play a role in affecting the child's neurological development prior to birth while they are still developing within the womb. Excessive exposure of the fetus to elevated levels of pro-inflammatory cytokines is an important contributing factor that might also determine the presence or level of severity of autism or other developmental disorders at the time of birth.

Sources of pro-inflammatory cytokine exposure during pregnancy may include intestinal bacterial imbalance of the mother, inadequate omega-3 and excessive omega-6 fatty acid dietary intake, exposure to tobacco smoke, urban air pollution, periodontal disease, as well as excessive dietary AGEs (advanced glycation end-products) intake.

After birth, excessive pro-inflammatory cytokines can disrupt a child's normal neuronal development and inhibit the brain from repairing commonplace injuries that occur from physical, emotional, chemical, and inflammatory trauma.

Improving Omega-3 Fatty Acid Transfer in the Third Trimester

During pregnancy the mother will transfer half of her entire omega-3 fatty acid stores to her child during the third trimester. This transfer provides the child with enough omega-3 fatty acids required for normal neurological development during their first year of life. This also signals how important the supply of omega-3 fatty acids are to healthy development.

The importance of omega-3 fatty acids is so significant that the child of a mother supplementing with high doses of omega-3 fatty acids from fish oil will give birth to a child with an I.Q. that is almost 10 points higher than they would have had if the mother did not supplement.

If the mother's diet is low in omega-3 fatty acids and high in inflammation-causing omega-6 fatty acids, the child may experience a similar imbalance of omega fatty acids during the third-trimester transfer. The omega fatty acid imbalance will further increase the inflammatory cytokine level within the mother and child and may further impair normal brain development in the child.

Supplementation with extra virgin olive oil is critical to reduce the inflammatory state of the mother even further during pregnancy. Extra virgin olive oil contains high amounts of an omega-9 fatty acid called oleic acid that helps block and reverse the inflammatory damage caused by excessive dietary omega-6 fatty acid intake, as well as saturated fatty acids such as palmitic acid.

I typically recommend that the expectant mothers under my care supplement with 2,000-3,000 mg of fish oil per day, and that they also consume 2 tablespoons of COOC-certified extra virgin olive oil. High intakes of fish and olive oil are routine in many regions of the Mediterranean and as a natural consequence are known to be safe during pregnancy.

Pregnant women should not take a high-concentration DHA fish oil (DHA mg. are greater than EPA mg.). The predominant intake omega-3 fatty acids during evolution from fish had much more EPA than DHA. Although uncertain if biologically important, a relatively higher EPA concentration fish oil should be consumed during pregnancy (EPA mg. are greater than DHA mg.) to help mimic our evolutionary exposure.

Improving Intestinal Bacterial Balance During Pregnancy

To improve intestinal balance during pregnancy, I recommend my patients supplement if needed with the over the counter prebiotic plant fiber inulin. Although not as effective as rifaximin, inulin may improve the intestinal symptoms of bacterial overgrowth such as diarrhea, heartburn, nausea, and cramping.

Intestinal balance treatment options during pregnancy are limited to just the inulin fiber. The use of the non-absorbable antibiotic rifaximin to rebalance the intestinal bacteria has not been adequately studied during pregnancy and is never to be recommended for use during pregnancy.

Considerations After Delivery

As long as the infant child is able to maintain the proper balance of intestinal bacteria, they predictably will not develop inflammation nor excessive propionic acid production that occurs only from bacterial overgrowth of the small intestine.

Bacterial overgrowth in a newborn infant potentially could occur if their intestinal bacteria are disrupted by spending time within the NICU or by receiving antibiotics prior to discharge.

Since reversing intestinal bacterial imbalance and restoring the omega-3 to omega-6 fatty acid balance reverses many of the key features in autism, managing these issues upfront may theoretically help prevent regressive autism from occurring in some children.

If there is any suspicion of bacterial overgrowth in the mother or older siblings (since they would also be colonized with the mother's bacterial blend of my patient, the younger sibling), I generally recommend supplementing the newborn infant with 1/32 to 1/16 tsp of powdered inulin fiber daily.

Fish oil and olive oil are not required since the additional omega fatty acids required from each of these will be provided though the mother's breast milk as long as she is taking each.

When the child is old enough to eat regular food, I recommend they be supplemented in addition with fish oil and that their food be cooked in COOC-certified extra virgin olive oil to protect them from toxic omega-6 fatty acids that will inevitably seep into their diet.

Considerations Specific to Vaccines

Personally, I support the vaccination of children. I am only against vaccinating children *when* they are actively experiencing bacterial overgrowth and *when* they still might have difficult recovering from an inflammatory surge due to unhealthy levels of pro-inflammatory cytokines within their brains.

As I have discussed in previous chapters, the brain can be injured through physical injury, emotional traumas, by chemical or toxic exposures, by the lack of oxygen, and though a surge of inflammatory chemicals called pro-inflammatory cytokines.

These pro-inflammatory cytokines are part of our natural repair process. These pro-inflammatory cytokines can be released under other common circumstances as well.

In animal studies surgeries of the abdomen or chest, fractures of the long bones, brain infections, and vaccines are all capable of disrupting brain function due to a release of pro-inflammatory cytokines.

It is important to note that when the pro-inflammatory cytokines injure the brain of a healthy mouse with a normal intestinal bacterial balance and normal omega fatty acid intakes, the mouse is capable of fully recovering from the inflammatory stress of the vaccine within a few weeks.

If a mouse has primed microglia and increased levels of pro-inflammatory cytokines from bacterial overgrowth, the mouse does not fully recover from the vaccine injury, and residual damage is left behind (see Cunningham papers in reference appendix).

The residual damage from unrepaired brain injury contributes to the cumulative brain injury that I have discussed elsewhere in this book.

Vaccinations are designed to mimic exposure to an infectious organism in order to create a protective inflammatory, immune reaction. For a vaccine to be effective, the inflammation it triggers is an essential part of the protective reaction.

But depending on the brain health of the person vaccinated, the inflammatory surge of pro-inflammatory cytokines from the vaccine may have unintended consequences such as the worsening of bacterial overgrowth, developmental delay, or may result in cumulative brain damage.

Knowing that autism and the associated developmental delay cannot generally occur without the elevated propionic acid levels and inflammation triggered by bacterial overgrowth of the small intestine, the unavoidable question becomes how might the inflammatory reaction from the vaccine increase the likelihood of autism, developmental disorders, or cumulative brain injury?

The debate has raged for decades over the direct and indirect consequences of vaccinations on the incidence of autism. My personal views of the possible role of vaccines in triggering autism are as follows.

The inflammatory surge commonly delivered by vaccines may be strong enough to even temporarily disrupt the function of the autonomic nervous system and can impair the function of the parasympathetic branch of the autonomic nervous system in particular. Impaired parasympathetic function is associated with slowed intestinal motility, a risk factor for the development or worsening of bacterial overgrowth. Slowing of intestinal peristalsis from other situations such as general anesthesia, abdominal surgery, concussions, and disorders such as scleroderma and renal failure are all associated with an increased risk in the development of bacterial overgrowth of the small intestine.

In my medical practice, I have witnessed the relapse of bacterial overgrowth from routine vaccination in both children and adult patients under my care. If a child acquires a mild form of bacterial overgrowth from their mother or from the use of antibiotics early in the course of their life, a subsequent vaccination might worsen bacterial overgrowth and might encourage the excessive production of propionic acid through its negative effect on peristalsis. Again, I personally support the vaccination of children. I am only against vaccinating children when they are experiencing bacterial overgrowth and when they have an unhealthy level of pro-inflammatory cytokines within their brains.

The issue then becomes when does a patient receive life-saving vaccinations that are necessary, and how might we improve the patient's health before and during such vaccination.

Vaccines are the only way to presently protect children from several deadly illnesses for which there is no other treatment. Vaccinations against measles and many other childhood illnesses have been an enormous success. Without vaccinations, massive epidemics will once again become the deadly norm.

As a reminder, there are no antibiotics to treat a child infected with measles, mumps, rubella, or polio.

Another important consideration is the timing of the vaccinations. I believe that delaying the vaccination of children for a few months until their intestinal bacteria and inflammatory status has been improved with inulin and omega-3 fatty acids from fish oil would predictably help their nervous systems to stabilize and should help to minimize the risk of developing autism, future developmental delay, and cumulative brain injury.

To explore possible preventative opportunities, I logically begin with the simple nutritional tools that impact existing autism and childhood disorders and I use them proactively by starting my infant or young child patient on daily inulin and fish oil supplementation.

Balancing the intestinal bacteria with 1/16 to 1/4 teaspoon of powdered inulin per day in my patient with suspected bacterial overgrowth has the potential to lessen the likelihood of bacterial overgrowth with propionic acid-producing bacteria from decreased peristalsis.

It is the sudden production of excessively high levels of propionic acid from the intestinal tract that saturate the child's brain and explain why some parents report that they witnessed their child appear to drift away in a stuporous state within in hours or days after receiving a vaccine. Excessive propionic acid production is the cause of the classic regressive autism scenario.

In addition, supplementing of omega-3 fatty acids from fish oil and cooking all foods in COOC-certified extra virgin oil olive should also help shift the phenotype of the microglia within the child's brain into the M2-microglia phenotype that are anti-inflammatory and help repair brain injuries.

Increasing the preponderance of repairing and anti-inflammatory M2-microglia should allow the child's brain to fully recover from any resulting inflammatory brain injury from the vaccine.

After roughly three to four months on protocol, I estimate the inflammation and microglial function should be improved enough from the inulin and oils to safely begin vaccination.

I readily admit that there are no "placebo-blinded human studies" to support my preventative recommendations contained in this chapter. My recommendations come from deductive reasoning and common sense that if inulin and fish oil can reverse the neurological damage underlying autism and developmental delay, then the same treatments stand a reasonable chance of preventing them as well.

Many children with autism and developmental issues under my care have gone forward and safely received vaccines using these recommendations.

But the reality we now face on a global level is that we suddenly have one or two generations of children who are experiencing increasing rates of autism and developmental disorders which until recently have been unexplained.

These children and others yet to be born need help, and I believe from the success I have seen using the simple nutritional tools of The Nemechek Protocol® that this is a preventative approach to be considered in the future as well.

21

SOMETIMES MIRACLES DO HAPPEN

TRUE STORIES OF RECOVERY

Microcephaly Plus Autism

Srihan is a nine-year-old boy who was adopted after spending the first five years of his life in an orphanage under extremely harsh conditions. To complicate matters, Srihan also had microcephaly, a condition with a small skull and smaller than a normal brain. Children with microcephaly often have associated developmental and intellectual delay. Srihan had severe receptive and expressive communication challenges and extreme aggression that required the use of the potent antipsychotic agent, risperidone.

Within the first year of The Nemechek Protocol® Srihan had subtle but significant gains, but he experienced inulin failure within about six months. Monthly cycles of rifaximin were having a very positive effect on his aggression. Still, before the end of each month, his intestinal bacterial overgrowth would relapse, and his aggression would increase again.

Starting continuous rifaximin was the key for Srihan. Within three months, his mother wrote to me stating his aggression was so greatly improved that he was now off risperidone entirely, and he was nearly off the clonidine that had been added for his anxiety.

Srihan can now verbally communicate when he is upset, and he even can ask his parents to help him calm down at times. He can watch a TV program for kids, interact appropriately with the program. He can answer the questions they ask the viewers correctly.

When prompted, he is now also able to slow down his non-stop chatter. Previously, he would ask what is for supper over and over all day, back-to-back questioning even after being told what was for supper. Now he says, "Not going to talk about it over and over, I will release it".

He has startled his teachers and therapists with his gains over the last several months. His gains were unexpected for a child with microcephaly, especially with autism, because of his small brain size. Srihan's mother said she gets notes from school almost every day about his miraculous improvements. She is excited about his future.

The Importance of Fish Oil and Olive Oil

Avery is a five-year-old girl with autism whose parents told me she was "started" on The Nemechek Protocol® eight months before our first visit. Her parents reported that Avery experienced a nice increase in awareness, better eye contact, and seemed more interested in interacting with her parents and younger brother. But despite these first few gains initially, she had no notable gains in comprehension, speech, or improvement in her hyperactivity.

Shortly into our first office consultation, I realized the problem was Avery hadn't been "started" on the protocol. She was only taking inulin. She had never taken any fish oil and olive oil. Her parents had fallen prey to the excitement of seeing an awakening after adding the inulin. Still, they had never really read the reasons why the fish oil and olive oil were both so essential for healing.

I prescribed the appropriate fish oil and olive oil for Avery. Within a few weeks, her father wrote excitedly to me about how many positive gains she showed after starting the oils. She was much more responsive and aware and had less toe-walking. She was still having tantrums, but they became less frequent and less intense. Now she can handle transitions (leave the park, leave home) without melting down emotionally.

Although I talk in this book about how important it is to balance the intestinal bacteria correctly, that is just one element of my protocol. This patient is a vivid reminder of how critical it is to have the proper doses and approved fish oil and olive oil brands because inulin alone will not allow full recovery.

Simply put, The Nemechek Protocol® requires balanced intestinal bacteria plus fish oil and olive oil, with vagus nerve stimulation added when incomplete recovery is observed.

Higher Phenol Counts can Help

The primary goal of The Nemechek Protocol® is to lower inflammation. If it is reduced enough, the body's natural repair and rejuvenation mechanisms become re-activated, and the body begins healing itself. All the individual components of the protocol can lower inflammation. Still, the anti-inflammatory properties of olive oil have only recently become more fully appreciated, and the following is a story that exemplifies this point.

Naomi is a young girl who had experienced a great deal of recovery with The Nemechek Protocol® and saw continual recovery from a wide array of developmental challenges except her hyperactivity. She was on the proper doses of fish oil and olive oil, getting five minutes of vagus nerve stimulation and monthly cyclic rifaximin. She was not experiencing a plateau as everything was slowly recovering except for her hyperactivity.

I did not need to increase her dose to continuous rifaximin. This would not help this situation because going from monthly cycles of rifaximin to continuous rifaximin was only helpful for a plateau when all aspects of recovery had stalled. In Naomi's case, everything else seemed to be recovering, just not her hyperactivity.

Her situation seemed to me like there was still a source of inflammation in her life interfering with her progress. I needed to lower her inflammation a little further. The sources of inflammation that I looked for included dental issues, chronic infections such as sinuses, and Vitamin D deficiency. Naomi had none of these issues, but her family reported using a COOC-certified brand of olive oil from a large chain store with an unknown phenol concentration. I had them switch her olive oil to a mid-range olive oil with a known phenol count of approximately 350.

After taking the new olive oil for a month, Naomi's mother reported that Naomi could sit longer during a meal and when working online. Her teachers also reported improvements when she was in class as well.

Although I think standard lower phenol count olive oils are adequate for most kids to use during recovery, in this case, presumably increasing the phenol to mid-range made a rapid change that Naomi's parents were hoping for.

Phenol Toxicity is Real

The story of excessive phenols is best told right after Naomi's story about increasing the phenols in her olive oil. Peter is an eight-year-old boy who had been on The Nemechek Protocol® for 15 months, and he was experiencing significant gains in receptive skills. He was learning to socialize with his brother, had started showing interest in speaking, and had been able to even say a few words.

After chatting with others on the internet, his mother switched his olive oil from a good quality COOC-certified brand to an ultra-high phenol concentrated olive oil with a total phenol count greater than 2,000. Within a few days of starting the ultra-high phenol olive oil, her son experienced his first seizure. That new brand of olive oil was stopped, and his seizures stopped for almost three months until his mother restarted the ultra-high phenol olive oil again. Once again, her son had his second seizure within a few days. I counseled his mother to never use an ultra-high phenol content olive oil again with her son.

His mother has fallen victim to the "more is better" logic that often fails in medicine. Phenols are not magical substances that have an unlimited ability to improve health. Phenols are, in fact, natural compounds that trigger what is known as hormetic stress. Hormetic stress, or hormesis, is a process that improves cellular function when cells are exposed to small amounts of a toxin. In the case of olive oil, the toxins are the phenols.

A more traditional olive oil phenol concentration in a Mediterranean diet (less than 600) creates positive hermetic stress and stimulates cells to repair and rejuvenate. But excessive amounts of phenols (>700) have been shown to cause damage in human cell cultures.

Peter is not the only patient under my care who has suffered seizures or had other neurological conditions worsened after switching to an ultra-high phenol count olive oil. While I understand the human impulse to give "more" and to try to rush healing, the rule of "more is better" often causes more problems medically. I do not recommend the use of any ultra-high phenol olive oils.

A History of Encephalomyelitis

Although our book focuses on children with autism and other forms of developmental delay, the protocol's ability to allow the nervous system to recover from other forms of neurological injury is unbelievable at times.

This story is about Ava. Up until the age of four, Ava was developing normally, but then disaster struck. Ava developed a mild fever followed by delirium, and she ultimately became comatose after two weeks. She was diagnosed with autoimmune encephalitis. She was treated with infusions of immune globulin and then plasmapheresis to get her immune system to stop attacking her brain.

By the time she came to see me at the age of seven, therapies had only been able to allow her to tolerate sitting upright for a few hours. She could only hold herself upright in a walker for a few minutes, and she was unable to walk. Her speech was limited to only a few individual words. She had severe constipation, and she still required a feeding tube. Her bladder problems and generally weak health required hospitalizations almost monthly because of urinary tract infections.

Ava was started on inulin, fish oil, and olive oil given through her feeding tube and once-daily vagus nerve stimulation. Within three months, her frequent hospitalizations had stopped. Her arms and hands' muscular contractions began to relax to the point she no longer required Botox injections. Her speech and general noise-making developed more inflections and tones. In the past, she had bilateral hip fractures, and now that she was on the protocol, she began getting more use and strength in her legs.

She was believed to be completely blind since her original hospitalization at age four. Still, a recent visual evoked potential test (a test of the visual pathway from the retina to the occipital cortex) indicated her vision might, in fact, be returning as well. As time progressed, her parents would catch Ava tracking them or one of her siblings as they moved around a room.

After a few more months, the parents and I decided to be more aggressive with her SIBO to maximize her recovery. We switched her from inulin to monthly cycles of rifaximin while continuing her fish oil, olive oil, and vagus nerve stimulation. At one point, her vagus nerve stimulator quit working, and her mother noted her stomach pains and vomiting began to return right away. Shortly after resuming her vagus nerve stimulator, her stomach pains and vomiting stopped.

As her muscle contractions stopped and her strength improved, Ava began walking using a walker. She had also regained enough movement of her hands to feed herself and was learning how to chew. Her ability to swallow was improved to such a degree she began maintaining most of her caloric intake by mouth instead of through her feeding tube.

Ava's vocalizations continue to improve. She can now say "mom" and other sounds such as "ish" along with a wide variety of very different tones, volumes, and lengths of phonation. All of these improvements have occurred in the nine months since starting the protocol.

Most recently, she can walk up the stairs to her bedroom without assistance. Ava continues to catch up to her peers in weight and height, her vision continues to improve, and she remains hospital-free.

Twice Daily Vagus Nerve Stimulation

Jerry is a fifteen-year-old boy who started The Nemechek Protocol® at the age of twelve. He had developed a rather severe degree of regressive autism shortly after his first birthday. He had some improvements on and off with various treatment efforts (ABA, speech, biomedical). Still, he did not realize significant and consistent gains until he started my protocol and graduated to monthly cycles of rifaximin.

After two years on monthly cycles of rifaximin along with fish oil, olive oil, and once-daily vagus nerve stimulation, he experienced dramatic improvements in comprehension, maturity, socialization, and speech. The only problem was that although he could answer questions and converse quite clearly and readily, he would only do so if others initiated the conversation. He seemed unable or unwilling to start a conversation.

At this point, he was essentially on the complete protocol for children (The Nemechek Protocol® for Adults has additional elements), and his conversational ability was the only aspect not improving. I decided to lower his inflammation even more by increasing his vagus nerve stimulation to two to three times per day.

Within two months, Jerry was described as a "chatterbox" who seemed to want to talk about many things. His parents were delighted, and his father said, "I sometimes wish he was a little quiet again, which makes me think he is now like typical for a happy teenager."

Aggressive Behavior

Jackson is a seventeen-year-old who regressed into autism around the age of two. As many kids do, he made some gains with continuous and long-term ABA and other therapies. Still, as he aged into his teen years, he became more and more aggressive and easily angered. Now that he was a grown man's size, his uncontrollable aggressive events put him and those around him at obvious risk. Jackson had tried on various medications to control his outbursts. Still, they all seemed to make his behavior even more erratic.

After his mother reading about the protocol on Facebook, she started The Nemechek Protocol® with fish oil, olive oil, and inulin gummies. She thought that he was more alert within a couple of days and seemed to genuinely be happier, something she had not seen in many years since the aggression began. His outbursts had dramatically declined within eight weeks, going from one or two events per day to only a few per month.

Unfortunately, as often happens in older children using inulin on the protocol, Jackson's angry and aggressive outbursts started to increase again. I felt it was because he once again had excessive bacteria colonizing his small intestine, a sure sign of inulin failure. Because of the potential danger his outbursts posed to him and those around him, the parents and I decided to skip trying monthly cycles of rifaximin and go straight to daily, continuous rifaximin. This turned out to be just the right decision for Jackson.

Within a few months, Jackson's speech was becoming increasingly audible and complex. He was beginning to show how intelligent he was with the type of questions he was asking. His unique personality was starting to show, as was his sense of humor. His newly developed impulse control allowed him to adapt to the changes the pandemic caused in his routine.

I am happy to report I saw Jackson again shortly before finishing this edition of the book. I am delighted to say he continues to improve, and his outbursts have entirely stopped. He is no longer stuck in obsessive loops, and his anxiety is better. His stimming behaviors are gone, and he is much more relaxed while socializing with familiar people. His parents report seeing more and more neurotypical features appearing every day. He is also excelling in school at a pace that has him rapidly catching up in math and reading skills. He has even started talking about having a girlfriend.

I am still amazed daily at how capable the nervous system is of recovery as long as you maintain the brain in a healthy, non-inflamed environment.

Better without ABA

James is a six-year-old boy with autism who had been on The Nemechek Protocol® for about eighteen months when the pandemic struck in the spring of 2020. Just like other schools, at James' school, his work with therapists was suspended.

While talking with his parents during one of our conversations, his parents were concerned that his recovery may come to a halt without the therapists' assistance. During the first spring of the pandemic, I had similar conversations with other parents whose autistic children also had their school and therapy sessions suspended.

A few months passed by, and I have another follow-up consultation with James' parents. They were surprised by the extent of his continued recovery in the absence of attending his formal therapy sessions. Not only had he continued to improve in his verbal communication, but he was now seeking out his younger brother to play. He had very quickly learned to ride his bicycle. Continued and even accelerated gains by children despite discontinuing therapy sessions were reported to me by many other parents.

None of this was much of a surprise to me. For several years, I have observed children with autism make fantastic gains once the intestinal bacteria have been rebalanced and the propionic acid stupor eliminated. My general feeling is that the ability to speak and socialize are genetically coded in our species, no different than birds knowing how to build a nest without being taught. Once inflammation is suppressed, and the brain's natural developmental process begins, speech and socialization will follow.

When schools began reopening in the fall of the same year, I was surprised at the number of parents reporting that their child's gains seemed to slow. In some cases, progress almost stopped once their prior therapies were re-introduced. This was not a blanket observation but was reported by a significant number of parents.

Given the varying circumstances, some children seemed to enjoy and benefit from their renewed therapy sessions. But clearly, others had gained enough awareness and sense of self-purpose that they no longer were willing to participate. Whether they found the sessions' repetitive nature tedious, dull, they were actively deciding not to participate.

Once children with autism and developmental issues begin their recovery, we need to re-assess if therapies previously are still necessary. I commonly encounter new patients enrolled in 30 to 40 hours of therapy per week. This is the equivalent of a full-time job for these children. Like adults who hate their job, they will not thrive in a similar unpleasant setting.

Rattlesnake Bite "Regression"

Managing plateaus and problems is difficult when your patient cannot tell you what wrong, what hurts is, or what happened. Some things that can trigger a plateau are a surprise to both the parents and me, so when all else fails, examine your child for hidden physical injuries.

Dallas is a thirteen-year-old non-verbal boy who had been on The Nemechek Protocol® for two years. He tolerated supplementation with inulin, fish oil, olive oil, and vagus nerve stimulation once a day. Dallas was missing some fish oil doses about every other day, so his progress was slow yet steady.

His parents reported that he had a sudden and severe regression with a great deal of anxiety. He was also making odd hissing noises and sounds like a snake. His parents examined him. Upon finding a set of puncture marks on his body, they sought immediate emergency medical attention. It was determined that Dallas had been bit by a rattlesnake while playing in his yard. He was unable to communicate his potential life-threatening injury to his parents.

During the time immediately after the bite, he did go through a brief phase where he bit himself and had increased defiance with his online school. Dallas did fully recover from the rattlesnake bite. He is almost able to speak, is capable of imaginative play, has better penmanship, and has learned to ride a bicycle.

Concussion Causing Monthly Rifaximin Failure

Anastasia is an eight-year-old girl with a history of autism marked by severe aggression episodes (road rage type). She would injure herself by biting her hand and pounding her head on the floor, and she had also started trying to bite her mother and her sister if they were nearby. These episodes began to improve after starting The Nemechek Protocol® with inulin. Still, after nine months, the inulin began to fail, and she hit a plateau. At this point, I started her on monthly, ten-day cycles of twice-daily rifaximin.

As I had hoped, the aggression episodes began declining in frequency and intensity. After 10 months, her aggression had subsided entirely, and she was experiencing solid gains in speech, motor function, and comprehension.

Last fall, Anastasia was running through the house, and she slipped and hit her head on a tile floor. She developed swelling and bruising on the injury site, and she was in obvious pain. She seemed to heal without incident and her behavior immediately following the injury was unchanged.

But about two weeks later, her mother began noticing that Anastasia's aggression and raging anger began to re-appear. She started screaming and crying for extended periods when nobody could console her. Her parents feared she might hurt herself from kicking her feet against walls and doors.

Typically, the noticeable change in behavior from a head injury occurs within a child within a few days, not two weeks later. A repeat CT scan of the head excluded the presence of a subdural hematoma, which is a bleed between the brain and the skull that can cause symptoms several weeks after an injury.

There were no other intervening issues such as a sinus infection, dental problems, or obvious psychological challenges that would account for her worsening behavior. I believed her angry outbursts were being caused by a relapse in her intestinal bacteria.

Trauma to the nervous system can slow the intestinal tract's motility, which increases the risk for recurrence of bacterial overgrowth. Because of the intestinal tract's slower motility, her bacterial overgrowth was relapsing even more rapidly, and her once-monthly course of rifaximin was not controlling the overgrowth. Her recurrence of angry outbursts was not directly from the brain injury jury but indirectly from the bacterial overgrowth in her small intestine.

Simply shifting Anastasia's rifaximin regimen from ten-day cycles to a non-stop, continuous regimen stopped her angry outbursts. I will transition her back down to her monthly, ten-day courses of rifaximin after maybe six months.

Worsening Behavior from Pain

Aarav is a ten-year-old boy I met in 2019 after being on some ingredients of The Nemechek Protocol® since 2018. Previously, he had been obsessed with keeping all doors and cabinets in his entire home closed. If any family member opened the door to enter or leave a room, he would screech, run towards the door and close it. If his mother or father needed to open or a kitchen cabinet, he would do the same and close it. His behaviors were so disruptive that the family removed the doors from the main living areas and removed all the cabinet fronts from the kitchen and the bathroom Aarav used.

After three to four months on the protocol, these behaviors had almost completely stopped. Some of the doors and cabinet fronts were able to be rehung. After eighteen months on the protocol, Aarav's comprehension had greatly improved. Aarav was now playing with his siblings, and his speech had grown to include a wide variety of words and strings of two-to-three-word sentences.

But suddenly, within about one week, his obsession with doors and cabinets needing to be closed returned. I learned that he had an ear infection, a situation that requires the use of antibiotics to clear the infection. There was more going on, and soon we learned how much a hidden source of inflammation was triggering his symptoms.

During the antibiotics, he also took Motrin (Ibuprofen) to control his pain and inflammation. While on the Motrin, his pelvic grinding and other behaviors subsided. When the Motrin dose was later reduced, the family noticed his pelvic grinding and headbanging behaviors returned.

We eventually discovered that Aarav also had a dental infection. We kept him on the Motrin until he could go to the dentist for his dental procedure. After undergoing minor dental surgery, I restarted his monthly, 10-day rifaximin courses. His behavior began to dramatically improve, and now he is back on track and making gains again.

Inflammation can disrupt progress in a child's recovery and can come from a variety of different sources.

PANS and Low Blood Pressure

Henri is a 17-year-old boy that had been diagnosed with PANS. Henri had an unremarkable childhood except for a few sports concussions in grade school, constipation, and minor anxiety. Henri experienced a rapid onset of symptoms (practically overnight) three years earlier. Some minor improvements were noted over the next year, followed by an even worse decline in the year before becoming my patient.

When I first met him, he had bacterial overgrowth symptoms such as intolerance to spices, tomatoes, and milk intolerances. He felt somewhat better after restricting his diet of gluten. He also experienced recurrent strep throat, needed to exercise to think clearly, had trouble sleeping, daytime fatigue, poor concentration, excessive thirst, and constantly tapped his feet or wiggled his legs. By the time of his first visit, he had taken approximately fifteen antibiotics or other medicines in the intervening years and was currently on seventeen daily supplements.

Henri was put on ten days of rifaximin, a long-term regimen of fish oil, olive oil, and five minutes of daily vagus nerve stimulation.

Common head injuries in children may damage the autonomic nervous system and decrease blood pressure in the brain, a condition known as cerebral hypoperfusion. If the child has relatively low to normal levels of inflammation, they can quickly repair the injury. But suppose the child is experiencing high levels of inflammation from bacterial overgrowth. In that case, residual damage from the injury will remain, resulting in lower than normal brain blood pressure.

Henri, like most children, experienced a few brain traumas, and the accumulating damage caused a significant decline in his brain pressure. I recommended placing him on midodrine to help boost brain pressure, and his symptoms improved considerably.

His low brain blood pressure symptoms were why he could think clearer if constantly moving, like exercising or pacing, tapping his feet and legs, or consuming liquid or foods containing salt or sugar.

Despite being a teenager, Henri was more aware after starting the protocol. He giggled and acted almost like a "drunken sailor" for a few days after starting his first round of rifaximin. He became aware of his OCD behavior, and he could express that he did not know why he did those things. He said he really did not remember going to school or having friends at school. He could recall details of grade school but had no clear memories of attending middle school.

Henri's SIBO relapsed so quickly, and I prescribed monthly cycles of rifaximin to control the relapses for one year. I was able to taper him entirely off his midodrine and, ultimately, the scheduled rounds of rifaximin. Henri attended advanced placement academic classes, learned to drive a car, got a girlfriend, and started riding his horse again.

The last time I talked to Henri, he was off all of his medications, and he told me that I was the first doctor that had ever truly helped him.

Tics and Loss of Speech and Motor Function

Stefano was a neurotypical high school football player who came to see me because of "ankle and leg pain." He had hurt his leg during football practice, and he had developed hypersensitive nerve pain.

Stefano was confined to a wheelchair at his first visit, exhibiting uncontrollable tics with flailing arm and leg movements. He could only verbally communicate with a few sounds like "muh-muh-muh" and "bub-bub-bub." His father explained that he had been a typical child until his football injury that had never fully healed.

He had been healing from his ankle injury until an alternative health care provider put him on over-the-counter probiotics for minor intestinal issues. Once on the probiotic, Stefano developed tics and lost the ability to walk and talk. He was unable to attend class and had seen various other doctors who were baffled by his decline. His parents were ultimately told this must be some sort of neurodegenerative issue that would only get worse.

I suspected the probiotic bacteria had highjacked his nervous system. I had his father stop Stefano's probiotic and start on a ten-day course of rifaximin, fish oil, and olive oil.

Twenty-six days later, his mother called to tell my wife Jean that he was fully recovered. In fact, he was "perfect." His mother said he had responded immediately to the protocol, and his tics had stopped. He was already walking, talking, and back to attending school again. Jean asked her to please send a video of Stefano so we could see it for ourselves. He was indeed fully recovered and had no lingering symptoms.

I added this story to highlight why I have simple, absolute rules for my patients, such as no probiotics or additional vitamins or supplements. If one supplement can take away a typical teenage athlete's ability to walk and talk, trigger tics and uncontrollable movements. Then one might also prevent healing or delay recovery child already experiencing autism or developmental delays.

Seizures Resolve

Grant is twenty-five with a history of autism, seizures, headaches, and past treatment for Giardia (a parasite) that worsened his intestinal problems and other symptoms.

Grant became my patient in 2019 and was placed on daily fish and olive oil and monthly rifaximin. Shortly after beginning his first course of rifaximin, he could eat a variety of foods and his constipation resolved. His headaches had not improved, but he was having wisdom teeth issues.

Once a day, vagus nerve stimulation was added after a month on the protocol, and his seizures stopped. Grant did great with good adherence to his fish oil, drinking two tablespoons of olive oil and cooking with olive oil and vagus nerve stimulation. He was still on a few supplements because his mother was very hesitant to give them up. Has not had any seizures since starting VNS. In the last few weeks, his intolerance for food and constipation resolved.

Four months later, he was still using his vagus nerve stimulator consistently and had no new seizures. Compliance with the protocol had slipped. His parents told me he was only taking his getting fish oil three or four days per week. They were still cooking with olive oil, but he no longer took the additional tablespoons of olive oil. He was having headaches again, and seasonal allergy issues had returned. I prescribed another 10-day course of rifaximin and urged daily compliance with the protocol ingredients.

Six months later and Grant was still using his vagus nerve stimulator and remained seizure-free. Unexpectedly his mother stopped his fish oil and EVOO and restarted his former supplements because he was having tooth pain. His headaches and allergies were worse, and his mother had also started giving him an additional homeopathic allergy medicine. Grant was still seizure-free, but now he had intense anxiety, and he was now having episodes of striking himself in the head.

Grant's wisdom teeth were extracted soon afterward, and his mother stopped the extra supplements and restarted The Nemechek Protocol®. Grant felt better almost immediately after starting rifaximin.

Two years later, Grant remains seizure-free and is consistent with the protocol. He can tolerate flying on an airplane now, is headache-free, and no longer self-injurious. We have reduced the rifaximin to as needed for intestinal disturbances. On days when he feels his anxiety building, he is treated with an additional five-minute session.

Autism, Down's Syndrome, and Low Muscle Tone

Jose is a nine-year-old with autism, Down's Syndrome, and low muscle tone and was placed on The Nemechek Protocol®. Before starting, he had no speech, had sensory and stimming behaviors, and had little interest in his family or his iPad. He had minimal reaction to his environment and would show no response even if he wet his pants.

His parents slowly began with inulin, fish oil, and cooking in olive oil. He started making some eye contact, pointing at things, and there was a slight decrease in his tantrums. Once he became my patient, I added a ten-day course of rifaximin because of his recent lack of progress from possible inulin failure.

His parents reported strict compliance with giving him his fish oil and olive oils. And as evidence, they brought a journal showing the exact minute of each day that he took the protocol ingredients. Such charting is not necessary or recommended, but it did demonstrate their commitment for their son to never miss a dose. Jose showed more interest in his environment and his iPad. Still, there was no change in his stimming behaviors of flapping his hands, waking at night, or road rage anger and outbursts.

At their four-month follow up I added once daily vagus nerve stimulation. Jose's therapist noted that he started making "excellent progress" in the months that followed. Jose's coordination improved, and he was attempting to make sounds. Although he still had road rage temper tantrums, they were decreasing in frequency and intensity.

Near the one-year point, I felt he was relapsing with SIBO more frequently than we realized, so I prescribed a twelve-month course of continuous rifaximin. During those twelve months, his coordination and muscle tone dramatically improved. Jose's attention span increased, and he began to sit longer for more extended periods and for non-preferred activity. He was attempting expressive speech. He could now do 20- and 30-piece puzzles, and he can type over 40 words on his iPad. His parents were still working on potty training, but now he would react if he wet his pants or spilled a glass, and he interacted with his family.

Jose presently is on monthly cycles of rifaximin, and his gains have steadily continued. For the first time ever, he was excited to open his Christmas gifts. His brain continues to heal and mature, and he now understands jokes, he can sing with his sister when she practices her singing lessons, and he has begun growing in both height and weight.

Stroke at Birth

Will is a six-year-old boy who experienced a large stroke at birth with damage to the left side of his brain. He had been treated with many antibiotics, took medicine for acid reflux, had impairments in speech, and was developmentally delayed. Then at age 2, he started showing characteristics of autism.

Will began The Nemechek Protocol® at age five with inulin, fish oil, and olive oil. Shortly before starting the protocol, he had a severe reaction to a mosquito bite, which left him acting very aggressive, hyperactive, and with self-injurious behaviors. His hyperactivity interrupted learning at school, and he was constantly jumping on the sofa or his bed. It made it nearly impossible for him to lay down to go to bed.

In January 2020, Will became my patient and traveled overseas to see me before the pandemic travel restrictions began. I treated him with a single dose of rifaximin, and his self-injurious behavior stopped. However, he still had hyperactivity and mild anxiety at bedtime. I also recommended once daily vagus nerve stimulation, and within the first month, his awareness of his surroundings significantly increased.

Will had been exhibiting some aggression a few hours after taking his fish oil at first, but within 1-2 months, he tolerated it with no problem. He had begun talking more, had more awareness, and was otherwise progressing nicely. Will came down with chickenpox. Will seemed to have more anxiety after this time, and I recommended starting monthly cycles of rifaximin. Still, after 3 rounds, it was apparent Will seemed to be subtly relapsing before the end of the cyclic.

By the fall of 2020, it was clear that his SIBO was relapsing at a rate that he needed continual rifaximin for a minimum of twelve months. Today Will continues to have better awareness, less hyperactivity, better sleep and continues to make gains. After completing twelve months of continuous rifaximin, we plan on reducing him to the ten-day monthly rifaximin dosing regimen.

Blowing Out a Birthday Candle

Colton was five years old when he started The Nemechek Protocol®. He had poor focus, developmental delay, little interest in his surroundings, a limited diet, and was completely non-verbal. He was started on inulin, fish oil, and olive oil. As his awareness increased, he became more interested in his home environment and even wanted to spend more time outdoors.

In the first few months, he began responding to his name and following one-step commands. He learned to say a few words like "mama" and "bye-bye" and "hello," but still had no meaningful language.

By the end of the first six months, his appetite improved ate a greater variety of foods, and there was no more undigested food in stool. His comprehension improved, and he could do two steps commands and recognize family members and visitors to his house. He still did not play with his toys and seemed to have more road rage aggression, and would sometimes pull his little sister's hair. I started him on once-daily vagus nerve stimulation, as well as cyclic rifaximin. His gains were steady, but it was apparent he was relapsing before the next round of rifaximin was due. Accordingly, I prescribed twelve months of continuous rifaximin.

By the end of the first year, Colton has shown many gains with his developmental delays. His speech has improved to complex sentences, and he is reading on his iPad. His fine motor function has improved considerably, and Colton could open and close doors and discovered he liked to lock them. His comprehension continues to improve, and he can understand complex games and puzzles, and he listens and follows directions. As his imagination grew, he learned to play appropriately with his sister and no longer was aggressive or pulled her hair.

Recently Colton had his first awareness of his own birthday. He was excited for his birthday to arrive and had finally learned how to blow out his birthday cake candles for the first time. He continues to see steady gains in all areas and transition to a regular school in the fall.

Deaf Since Birth

Grace is a 28-year-old who had slipped into autism around the age of two. She had been deaf since birth and had significant developmental delay. She could do some sign language but had trouble moving her hands, and she had motor and balance issues. She often spilled foods and beverages and seemed unaware that she had done those things, never cleaning up her mess. She often "zoned out" and was unresponsive. She was tiny for her age, weighing about 70 pounds, with many food intolerances and an intense fear of eating any green food.

Her parents placed her on inulin and fish oil and discontinued the probiotics that she had taken for years. Her parents brought her to see me as she had recently started reacting to noises. Her whole life, she had never responded to noises. Still, there was no anatomical reason for her deafness, so they wanted to try rifaximin due to her age.

I prescribed a ten-day course of rifaximin, and she was treated intermittently through the first year. During that year, Grace had significant improvement in her communication skills; she started making sounds and then say words and learned to use a letter board. She began to respond to people with a combination of verbal and written responses, and she no longer needed to watch their lips to understand what they were saying to her.

Her food intolerance resolved, she was no longer afraid of green food and began to gain weight and even grow taller (I know this isn't supposed to happen at this age). Her balance and walking improved. She had more energy, less anxiety, and more calmly transitioned when leaving her home. She began setting the table for dinner, making drinks for everyone, cleaning up spills, and refilling water glasses during meals.

Grace was just one of several of my patients who experienced an improvement in their hearing. Others have similarly reported improved vision or finally developed a sense of smell as young adults. Although Grace's parents were delighted with her progress, they opted not to add vagus nerve stimulation to try to expand her present level of recovery.

22

HOPE IS ON THE HORIZON

The human brain has an enormous capacity for repair and rejuvenation. The microglia within the brain are proving to be capable of restarting their task of synaptic-neuronal pruning even after many years of being in a state of inflammatory paralysis.

The substantial reduction of pro-inflammatory cytokines within the brain is all that is necessary for the normal process of maturation and brain repair to begin anew.

We are also beginning to understand that once human genes are turned on by inflammation, they can ultimately be shut off again once the inflammatory environment within the body is significantly reduced.

My advice is the same for all my patients and their parents. Do your best to be patient, to give The Nemechek Protocol® and my overall approach to lower inflammation a chance, and to adopt a marathon mindset because brain recovery takes time and effort.

Because the path to recovery for many medical conditions is often five steps forward, and then sometimes one or two steps backward, we compare today's behavior to a child's behavior that was months or years earlier.

Comparing today to yesterday will only serve to put parents on an emotional roller coaster, and it could possibly lead parents to make some incorrect decisions for their child. The neurons within the human brain, like the growing of your hair, can only grow and change so fast.

Once the inflammation is suppressed, I believe that all that is required for continued recovery is a good solid inflammation suppressing regimen and patience. Remember, the neurons within the human brain, like your hair, grow slowly and therefore your child's improvement will occur slowly but steadily.

APPENDIX

NEMECHEK PROTOCOL-APPROVED BRANDS

Inulin

- Nemechek Blue Organic Inulin - available at NemechekBlue.com
- NOW Foods Inulin - available at multiple retail outlets and online retailers
- Fiber Choice®
- Phillips' ® Fiber Good® Gummies

Fish Oil

- Nordic Naturals Ultimate Omega in liquid or capsule form - available at multiple retail outlets and online retailers
- NOW Foods DHA-500 - available at multiple retail outlets and online retailers

Extra Virgin Olive Oil (EVOO)

- Nemechek Gold EVOO - available at NemechekGold.com
- Other COOC-certified EVOO brands - a listing is available at COOC.com

DOSING REFERENCE GUIDE

Dosing Information for Children:

I recommend starting all the ingredients at the same time or as soon as they become available. A modification approach is to start the children on just the fish and olive oils for the first 4 weeks and then start the inulin or rifaximin. The delay will allow the oils to fully saturate the brain and be ready to assist in the recovery once the intestine overgrowth is reversed with either inulin or rifaximin.

Ingredient #1 – Daily Extra Virgin Olive Oil Dosage

Use only COOC-certified and give raw uncooked olive oil daily either straight like medicine or mixed in food or drink. The minimal amount of olive oil is listed below.

- If under 4 years of age, give ¼-½ of a teaspoon (1.25-2.5 ml) of EVOO daily
- If 4 to 8 years old, give 1 teaspoon (5 ml) of EVOO daily
- If 9 to 12 years old, give 2 teaspoons (10 ml) of EVOO daily
- If 13 to 17 years old, give 1 tablespoon (15 ml) of EVOO daily
- If 18 years or older, give 2 tablespoons (30 ml) of EVOO daily

Ingredient #2 – Liquid Fish Oil Dosage

- Use the liquid form of fish oil produced by Nordic Natural called Ultimate Omega (NNUO)

- If under 4 years of age, give a 1/8 teaspoon (0.6 ml) of fish oil daily
- If 3 to 5 years old, give a 1/4 teaspoon (1.25 ml) of fish oil daily
- If 6 to 10 years old, give a 1/2 teaspoon (2.5 ml) of fish oil daily
- If 11 to 14 years old, give 1 teaspoon (5 ml) of fish oil daily or 2-3 DHA-500 tablets (NOW Foods)
- If 15 to 17 years old, give 2 teaspoons (10 ml) of fish oil daily or 4-5 DHA-500 tablets (NOW Foods)
- If 18 years or older, give 1 tablespoon (15 ml) of fish oil daily or 6 DHA-500 tablets (NOW Foods)

Ingredient #3 – Balance Intestinal Bacteria

Inulin and the prescription medication rifaximin (Xifaxan®) are two options to balance the intestinal bacteria. Starting with inulin is preferred in younger children while starting with rifaximin is recommended in older children because inulin is less effective in older children.

Choosing Between Inulin versus Rifaximin

- If under 8 years of age, use inulin to balance intestine bacteria
- If 8-14 years old, you can start with either inulin or rifaximin
- If 15 years of age or older, I recommend starting with rifaximin

Inulin Dosage

- Give a 1/8 teaspoon of powdered inulin (NOW Foods, Inc) once daily
- Can be mixed in food or drink
- Dosage does not change with age

Rifaximin (Xifaxan®) Dosage

- 550 mg twice daily for 10 days for ages five years and older
- Since the medication is not absorbed into the bloodstream, the dosage does not need to be adjusted for children 5-years-old and older.
- Medication can be crushed and mixed with food or drink if necessary
- This is a prescription medication and must be obtained through your physician

Notes on Adjusting the Inulin Dosage

As inulin reverses the bacterial overgrowth, the amount of propionic acid declines. Declining propionic acid levels leads to the awakening in which the child is more alert and cognizant of their surroundings.

If the initial dose of inulin does not trigger an "awakening" (more engaged, better eye contact, more aware of the world around them) then you may need to increase inulin slowly but do not exceed the ½ tsp dose. In my practice, I have not found that if a dose beyond ½ tsp produces meaningful results and I simply move on to Rifaximin.

Autistic children older than 10 and children who are not on the spectrum may not experience the "awakening". This does not mean that the protocol is not working.

Beyond just suppressing the production of propionic acid, the only true way to determine if the inulin is controlling the inflammatory stress produced by bacterial overgrowth is by observing improvements in the child's behavior and developmental issues over the ensuing 3 months.

If behaviors and neurological functions begin to improve, stay on this dose of inulin. If there is little to no improvement, the inulin is ineffective, and I recommend switching to monthly cycles of rifaximin.

Dosing Information for Adults (with and without Autism):

Ingredient #1 – Daily Extra Virgin Olive Oil (EVOO) Dosage

- Consume 30 ml (2 tablespoons) or more of EVOO per day
- Use only COOC-certified (California Olive Oil Certified) EVOO
- Olive oil should be raw and uncooked
- Can be mixed with food or drink

Ingredient #2 – Omega-3 Fatty Acids (EPA and DHA) from Fish Oil

- Adult patients require 3,000 mg of DHA daily. Although important, relatively little EPA penetrates the central nervous system and dosing is based upon the DHA fraction within the fish oil
- **Option 1** – Take 6 DHA-500 fish oil capsules (NOW Foods, Inc) per day
- **Option 2** – Take 15 ml (1 tablespoon) of Nordic Naturals Ultimate Omega liquid fish oil per day
- Either choice of fish oil may be taken with or without food, as a single dose or split into 2 doses

Ingredient #3 - Omega-3 Fatty Acids (ALA) from Nuts, Flax, or Chia

- **Option 1** – Consume a ¼ cup of nuts per day (almonds, pecans, pistachios, cashews, and walnuts)
- **Option 2** - Consume flax or chia seeds: 1/2 to 1 tablespoon per day.
- **Option 3** - Consume liquid flax oil: 500 to 1,000 mg once daily.

Ingredient #4 – Balance Intestinal Bacteria with Rifaximin

- Take 550 mg of rifaximin twice daily (in AM and PM) for 10 days
- Medication can be crushed and mixed with food or drink if necessary
- This is a prescription medication and must be obtained through your physician
- Repeated cycles of rifaximin may be required whenever the associated-intestinal symptoms return.

Ingredient # 5 – Vagal Nerve Stimulation

The purpose of vagus nerve stimulation in The Nemechek Protocol® is to suppress systemic and central nervous system inflammation. Lowering inflammation allows the nervous system to recover.

- Children and adults less than thirty years of age require only five minutes of continuous transcutaneous vagus nerve stimulation tVNS) per day
- At the proper settings, five minutes of tVNS is enough to significantly reduce inflammation throughout the body for at least 24 hours
- Between the ages of thirty and forty, five minutes of daily tVNS may not be enough and stimulation time may need to increase to one to two hours per day
- Patients over forty years of age almost universally need two hours of cycling tVNS

GLOSSARY

A Short Glossary of Scientific Terms

• **ALA, Alpha-Linolenic Acid** - An omega-3 fatty acid commonly supplemented in the form of nuts, flax, or chia.

• **Arachidonic Acid** - An omega-6 fatty acid that is part of the inflammation-producing process.

• **Autonomic Nervous System** - A large portion of the nervous system that regulates blood pressure, coordinates all organs (heart, intestines, bladder, etc.), controls inflammation, and regulates hormone production.

• **Bacterial Overgrowth** - Often used to refer to excessive bacterial growth within a segment of the intestinal tract. Less specific than the term SIBO which also implies a positive methane or hydrogen breath test or an abnormal quantification study from the small intestinal aspirate.

• **CBI** - Cumulative Brain Injury. The cumulative damage that results from the residual defects remaining after improperly repaired physical, inflammatory, or metabolic damage.

•**Concussion** - A physical injury to the brain that results in persistent symptoms for several days. Also referred to as a minor traumatic brain injury or mTBI.

•**Cumulative Brain Injury** - The cumulative damage that results from the residual defects remaining after improperly repaired physical, inflammatory, or metabolic damage.

•**Cytokines, Anti-Inflammatory** - Chemicals released from white blood cells that decrease the inflammatory response.

•**Cytokines, Pro-Inflammatory** - Chemicals released from white blood cells that increase the inflammatory response.

•**Developmental Delay** - The slowing of the normal rate of neurological and emotional maturation of a child. Often the result of excessive inflammation, nutritional deficiencies, and improper neuronal pruning.

•**Developmental Arrest** - The complete stoppage of the neurological and emotional maturation of a child. Often the result of excessive inflammation, nutritional deficiencies, and improper neuronal pruning.

•**DHA** - Docosahexaenoic acid (DHA) is an omega-3 fatty acid that is a primary structural component of the human brain, cerebral cortex, skin, and retina. Dietary sources include wild fish, fish oil, and meat from animals that feed on their natural food (e.g., grass-fed beef).

•**Digestive Enzymes** - Supplements often provided to improve digestion and intestinal symptoms.

•**Dysbiosis** - Refers to a general disruption of normal microbial balance within the intestinal tract. Dysbiosis can refer to any segment of the intestinal tract (mouth, small intestine, or colon), and although usually implies bacteria, may also be used in regard to protozoan, fungi, or archaebacteria.

•**EPA** - Eicosapentaenoic acid (EPA) is an omega-3 fatty acid. Dietary sources include wild fish, fish oil, and meat from animals that feed on their natural food (e.g., grass-fed beef).

•**EVOO** - Extra Virgin Olive Oil. EVOO is the highest quality of olive oil and is considered to have favorable flavor characteristics. It contains oleic acid which is an omega-9 fatty acid.

•**Inflammation** - A normal response by the immune system to fight infection or repair damaged tissues. Excessive inflammation can lead to damaging effects on the body.

•**Intestinal Bacterial Overgrowth** - Often used when referring to the excessive presence of bacteria within the small intestine. These bacteria often originate in the colon (lower or large intestine) and abnormally migrate up to the small intestine.

•**Inulin** - A prebiotic plant fiber derived from agave, onions, garlic, chicory is preferentially digested by the types of bacteria that normally inhabit the small intestine.

•**Linolenic Acid** - An omega-6 fatty acid that is part of the inflammation-producing process. Commonly found in plants and in high concentrations within a wide variety of cooking oils.

•**Microglia, Mo** - These are a specialized form of white blood cells that live in the brain. They are often referred to as surveillance or pruning microglia.

•**Microglia, M1** - These are a specialized form of white blood cells that live in the brain. They promote inflammation and are part of the healthy repair process but can cause damage if they become primed.

•**Microglia, M2** - These are a specialized form of white blood cells that live in the brain. They shut off inflammation and are part of the healthy repair process.

•**Microglia, Primed** - These are microglia that permanently morph into M1-microglia and prevent the brain from fully repairing brain trauma. They also are a major source of inflammatory cytokines within the brain.

•**mTBI** - Minor (lower case letter M) traumatic brain injury. A brain injury that is relatively mild and is commonly referred to as a concussion.

•**MTBI** - Major (upper case letter M) traumatic brain injury. A brain injury that is cause significant cellular damage and is often associated with intracranial bleeding.

•**Neuron** - A cell within the brain that carries or stores neurological information.

•**Neuroplasticity** - The process through which the brain develops new neuronal pathways to perform certain tasks.

•**Oleic Acid** - An omega-9 fatty acid that is very plentiful in olive oil. Oleic acid blocks the brain damage that can result from excessive omega-6 fatty acids and palmitic acid.

•**Omega-3 Fatty Acid** - These nutrients are unsaturated fatty acids and are important for normal metabolism. They are classified as an essential nutrient because humans are unable to synthesize omega-3 fatty acids and require them in their diet in order to remain healthy.

•**Omega-6 Fatty Acid** - These nutrients are a family of pro-inflammatory and anti-inflammatory polyunsaturated fatty acids. They are commonly found in plants and are classified as essential nutrients.

•**Omega-9 Fatty Acid** - These are unsaturated fatty acids and are not essential nutrients. Oleic acid found within olive oil is one example of an omega-9 fatty acid.

•**Palmitic Acid** - This nutrient is the most common saturated fatty acid found in animals, plants, and microorganisms. Excessive amounts in the diets of humans results in increase inflammation within the brain.

•**Phenotype** - The phenotype is the visible characteristic of how an animal, cell, or plant looks or behaves. (Genotype is the potential characteristic coded in the organism's DNA).

•**Prebiotic** - A form of fiber that induces the growth or activity of beneficial microorganisms (e.g., bacteria and fungi). The most common example is in the gastrointestinal tract where the digestion of prebiotic fibers can alter the composition of organisms in the gut microbiome.

•**Probiotic** - Bacterial organisms that are ingested or added to foods and are potentially beneficial to health.

•**Propionic Acid** = A small chain fatty acid produced by bacteria within the intestinal tract.

•**RifaGut™** - Another market brand name for rifaximin.

•**Rifaximin** - The generic term for the non-absorbable antibiotic sold under the brand name Xifaxan™, Rifagut™, Rifaximina™, and SIBOFix™.

•**SIBO** = Small Intestine Bacterial Overgrowth. A specific form of bacterial overgrowth that is designated by a positive methane or hydrogen breath test or an abnormal quantification study from a small intestinal aspirate.

•**SIBOFix™** - Another market brand name for rifaximin.

•**Synapse** - A portion of a neuron (or nerve cell) that permits the neuron to pass an electrical or chemical signal to another neuron.

•**The Nemechek Protocol®** - a medical treatment program invented by Dr. Patrick M. Nemechek, D.O. relating to methods for preventing, reducing, or reversing acute and/or chronic autonomic damage by the suppression of pro-inflammatory cytokines which is useful in treating a variety of diseases or conditions (U.S. Patent No. 10,335,356).

•**Toxic Encephalopathy** - The medical state of a child whose brain has essentially been drugged with excessive propionic acid.

•**Traumatic Brain Injury, TBI** - The focal term for a physical injury to the head and results in symptoms lasting more than 24 hours. See mTBI and MTBI.

•**Vagus Nerve** - The 10th cranial nerve of the human body that carries the signals in the parasympathetic branch of the autonomic nervous system.

•**Vagus Nerve Stimulation, VNS** - This is a medical treatment that involves delivering electrical impulses to the vagus nerve in the autonomic nervous system. Therapeutically VNS reduces inflammation throughout the brain and body and is capable of inducing neuroplasticity.

•**White Blood Cells (WBC)** - Cells of the immune system are often referred to as white blood cells or WBCs.

•**Xifaxan^{TM}** - This is the brand name of a time-released formulation of rifaximin sold within the United States.

SCIENTIFIC REFERENCES

We have provided a sampling of the many research articles that have helped shape the development of The Nemechek Protocol®.

Autonomic Dysfunction:

Taylor EC, Livingston LA, Callan MJ, Ashwin C, Shah P. Autonomic dysfunction in autism: The roles of anxiety, depression, and stress. Autism. 2021 Jan 24:1362361320985658. doi: 10.1177/1362361320985658. Epub ahead of print. PMID: 33491461.

Kong X, Liu J, Liu K, Koh M, Tian R, Hobbie C, Fong M, Chen Q, Zhao M, Budjan C, Kong J. Altered Autonomic Functions and Gut Microbiome in Individuals with Autism Spectrum Disorder (ASD): Implications for Assisting ASD Screening and Diagnosis. J Autism Dev Disord. 2021 Jan;51(1):144-157. doi: 10.1007/s10803-020-04524-1. PMID: 32410097.

Thapa R, Pokorski I, Ambarchi Z, Thomas E, Demayo M, Boulton K, Matthews S, Patel S, Sedeli I, Hickie IB, Guastella AJ. Heart Rate Variability in Children With Autism Spectrum Disorder and Associations With Medication and Symptom Severity. Autism Res. 2021

Jan;14(1):75-85. doi: 10.1002/aur.2437. Epub 2020 Nov 22. PMID: 33225622.

Baumann C, Rakowski U, Buchhorn R. Omega-3 Fatty Acid Supplementation Improves Heart Rate Variability in Obese Children. Int J Pediatr. 2018 Feb 26;2018:8789604. doi: 10.1155/2018/8789604. PMID: 29681953; PMCID: PMC5846363.

Hiura M, Nariai T, Sakata M, Muta A, Ishibashi K, Wagatsuma K, Tago T, Toyohara J, Ishii K, Maehara T. Response of Cerebral Blood Flow and Blood Pressure to Dynamic Exercise: A Study Using PET. Int J Sports Med. 2018 Feb;39(3):181-188. doi: 10.1055/s-0043-123647. Epub 2018 Jan 22. PMID: 29359277.

Bjørklund G. Cerebral hypoperfusion in autism spectrum disorder. Acta Neurobiol Expo (Wars). 2018;78(1):21-29. https://www.ncbi.nlm.nih.gov/pubmed/29694338

Goodman B. Autonomic Dysfunction in Autism Spectrum Disorders (ASD). *Neurology* April 5, 2016 vol. 86 no. 16 Supplement P5.117. http://www.neurology.org/content/86/16_Supplement/P5.117

Anderson CJ et al. Pupil and Salivary Indicators of Autonomic Dysfunction in Autism Spectrum Disorder. *Developmental psychobiology.* 2013;55(5):10.1002/dev.21051. https://www.ncbi.nlm.nih.gov/pmc/articles/PMC3832142/

Goodman B et al. Autonomic Nervous System Dysfunction in Concussion. *Neurology* February 12, 2013 vol. 80 no. 7 Supplement P01.265. http://www.neurology.org/content/80/7_Supplement/P01.265

La Fountaine MF. et al. Autonomic Nervous System Responses to Concussion: Arterial Pulse Contour Analysis. *Frontiers in Neurology* 7 (2016): 13. https://www.ncbi.nlm.nih.gov/pmc/articles/PMC4756114/

Amhed K. Assessment of Autonomic Function in Children with Autism and Normal Children Using Spectral Analysis and Posture Entrainment: A Pilot Study. *J of Neurology and Neuroscience.* 2015. Vol. 6 No. 3:37. http://www.jneuro.com/neurology-neuroscience/assessment-

of-autonomic-function-in-children-with-autism-and-normal-
children-using-spectral-analysis-and-posture-entrainment-a-pilot-
study.pdf

Bacterial Overgrowth:

Santos ANDR, Soares ACF, Oliveira RP, Morais MB. THE IMPACT OF SMALL INTESTINAL BACTERIAL OVERGROWTH ON THE GROWTH OF CHILDREN AND ADOLESCENTS. Rev Paul Pediatr. 2020 Jan 13;38:e2018164. doi: 10.1590/1984-0462/2020/38/2018164. PMID: 31939507; PMCID: PMC6958541.

Hoog CM, Lindberg G, Sjoqvist U. Findings in patients with chronic intestinal dysmotility investigated by capsule endoscopy. BMC Gastroenterol. 2007 Jul 18;7:29. doi: 10.1186/1471-230X-7-29. PMID: 17640373; PMCID: PMC1940016.

Wang L, Yu YM, Zhang YQ, Zhang J, Lu N, Liu N. Hydrogen breath test to detect small intestinal bacterial overgrowth: a prevalence case-control study in autism. Eur Child Adolesc Psychiatry. 2018 Feb;27(2):233-240. doi: 10.1007/s00787-017-1039-2. Epub 2017 Aug 10. PMID: 28799094.

Liu Z, Mao X, Dan Z, Pei Y, Xu R, Guo M, Liu K, Zhang F, Chen J, Su C, Zhuang Y, Tang J, Xia Y, Qin L, Hu Z, Liu X. Gene variations in autism spectrum disorder are associated with alteration of gut microbiota, metabolites and cytokines. Gut Microbes. 2021 Jan-Dec;13(1):1-16. doi: 10.1080/19490976.2020.1854967. PMID: 33412999; PMCID: PMC7808426.

Roussin L, Prince N, Perez-Pardo P, Kraneveld AD, Rabot S, Naudon L. Role of the Gut Microbiota in the Pathophysiology of Autism Spectrum Disorder: Clinical and Preclinical Evidence. Microorganisms. 2020 Sep 7;8(9):1369. doi: 10.3390/microorganisms8091369. PMID: 32906656; PMCID: PMC7563175.

MartÍn-Masot R, Molina Arias M, Diaz Martin JJ, Cilleruelo Pascual ML, Gutierrez Junquera C, Donat E, Román Riechmann E, Navas-

López VM. Management of small intestinal bacterial overgrowth by paediatric gastroenterologists in Spain. Rev Esp Enferm Dig. 2020 Dec 29. doi: 10.17235/reed.2020.7582/2020. Epub ahead of print. PMID: 33371710.

Avelar Rodriguez D, Ryan PM, Toro Monjaraz EM, Ramirez Mayans JA, Quigley EM. Small Intestinal Bacterial Overgrowth in Children: A State-Of-The-Art Review. Front Pediatr. 2019 Sep 4;7:363. doi: 10.3389/fped.2019.00363. PMID: 31552207; PMCID: PMC6737284.

Adams JB et al. Gastrointestinal flora and gastrointestinal status in children with autism -- comparisons to typical children and correlation with autism severity. *BMC Gastroenterology*. 2011. https://www.ncbi.nlm.nih.gov/pubmed/21410934

Wang L. Hydrogen breath test to detect small intestinal bacterial overgrowth: a prevalence case control study in autism. *Eur Child Adolesc Psychiatry*. 2017 Aug 10. https://www.ncbi.nlm.nih.gov/pubmed/28799094

Hsiao EY et al. The microbiota modulates gut physiology and behavioral abnormalities associated with autism. *Cell*. 2013;155(7):1451-1463. https://www.ncbi.nlm.nih.gov/pmc/articles/PMC3897394/

Cryan JF et al. Mind-altering microorganisms: the impact of the gut microbiota on brain and behaviour. *Nat Rev Neurosci*. 2012 Oct;13(10):701-12. https://www.ncbi.nlm.nih.gov/pubmed/22968153

Cao X, Liu K, Liu J, Liu YW, Xu L, Wang H, Zhu Y, Wang P, Li Z, Wen J, Shen C, Li M, Nie Z, Kong XJ. Dysbiotic Gut Microbiota and Dysregulation of Cytokine Profile in Children and Teens With Autism Spectrum Disorder. Front Neurosci. 2021 Feb 10;15:635925. doi: 10.3389/fnins.2021.635925. PMID: 33642989; PMCID: PMC7902875.

Cumulative Brain Injury:

Chang HK, Hsu JW, Wu JC, Huang KL, Chang HC, Bai YM, Chen TJ, Chen MH. Traumatic Brain Injury in Early Childhood and Risk of Attention-Deficit/Hyperactivity Disorder and Autism Spectrum

Disorder: A Nationwide Longitudinal Study. J Clin Psychiatry. 2018 Oct 16;79(6):17m11857. doi: 10.4088/JCP.17m11857. PMID: 30403445.

Bjørklund G, Kern JK, Urbina MA, Saad K, El-Houfey AA, Geier DA, Chirumbolo S, Geier MR, Mehta JA, Aaseth J. Cerebral hypoperfusion in autism spectrum disorder. Acta Neurobiol Exp (Wars). 2018;78(1):21-29. PMID: 29694338.

Cunningham C. Microglia and neurodegeneration: the role of systemic inflammation. *J Neurosci.* 2013 Mar 6;33(10):4216-33. https://www.ncbi.nlm.nih.gov/pubmed/22674585

Bilbo S, Stevens B. Microglia: The Brain's First Responders. Cerebrum. 2017 Nov 1;2017:cer-14-17. PMID: 30210663; PMCID: PMC6132046.

Olsen AB, Hetz RA, Xue H, Aroom KR, Bhattarai D, Johnson E, Bedi S, Cox CS Jr, Uray K. Effects of traumatic brain injury on intestinal contractility. Neurogastroenterol Motil. 2013 Jul;25(7):593-e463. doi: 10.1111/nmo.12121. Epub 2013 Apr 2. PMID: 23551971; PMCID: PMC3982791.

Wager-Smith, Karen, and Athina Markou. Depression: A Repair Response to Stress-Induced Neuronal Microdamage That Can Grade into a Chronic Neuroinflammatory Condition?*Neuroscience and biobehavioral reviews* 35.3 (2011): 742–764. https://www.ncbi.nlm.nih.gov/pubmed/208837188

Histamine:

Collins S, Reid G. Distant Site Effects of Ingested Prebiotics. *Nutrients.* 2016;8(9):523. https://www.ncbi.nlm.nih.gov/pmc/articles/PMC5037510/

Visciano P et al. Biogenic Amines in Raw and Processed Seafood. *Frontiers in Microbiology.* 2012;3:188. https://www.ncbi.nlm.nih.gov/pmc/articles/PMC3366335/

Feng c et al. Histamine (Scombroid) Fish Poisoning: a Comprehensive Review. *Clin Rev Allergy Immunol.* 2016 Feb;50(1):64-9. https://www.ncbi.nlm.nih.gov/pubmed/25876709

Jin X et al. Increased intestinal permeability in pathogenesis and progress of nonalcoholic steatohepatitis in rats. *World Journal of Gastroenterology : WJG.* 2007;13(11):1732-1736. https://www.ncbi.nlm.nih.gov/pubmed/17461479

Guo Y et al. Functional changes of intestinal mucosal barrier in surgically critical patients. *World Journal of Emergency Medicine.* 2010;1(3):205-208.   https://www.ncbi.nlm.nih.gov/pmc/articles/PMC4129678/
Inflammation:
Jafari A, de Lima Xavier L, Bernstein JD, Simonyan K, Bleier BS. Association of Sinonasal Inflammation With Functional Brain Connectivity. JAMA Otolaryngol Head Neck Surg. 2021 Apr 8. doi: 10.1001/jamaoto.2021.0204. Epub ahead of print. PMID: 33830194.

Zengeler KE, Lukens JR. Innate immunity at the crossroads of healthy brain maturation and neurodevelopmental disorders. Nat Rev Immunol. 2021 Jan 21. doi: 10.1038/s41577-020-00487-7. Epub ahead of print. PMID: 33479477.

Li YJ, Zhang X, Li YM. Antineuroinflammatory therapy: potential treatment for autism spectrum disorder by inhibiting glial activation and restoring synaptic function. CNS Spectr. 2020 Aug;25(4):493-501. doi: 10.1017/S1092852919001603. Epub 2019 Oct 29. PMID: 31659946.

Coomey R, Stowell R, Majewska A, Tropea D. The Role of Microglia in Neurodevelopmental Disorders and their Therapeutics. Curr Top Med   Chem.   2020;20(4):272-276.   doi: 10.2174/1568026620666200221172619.   PMID: 32091337;   PMCID: PMC7323119.

Mottahedin A, Ardalan M, Chumak T, Riebe I, Ek J, Mallard C. Effect of Neuroinflammation on Synaptic Organization and Function in the Developing Brain: Implications for Neurodevelopmental and

Neurodegenerative Disorders. Front Cell Neurosci. 2017 Jul 11;11:190. doi: 10.3389/fncel.2017.00190. PMID: 28744200; PMCID: PMC5504097.

Madore C, Leyrolle Q, Lacabanne C, Benmamar-Badel A, Joffre C, Nadjar A, Layé S. Neuroinflammation in Autism: Plausible Role of Maternal Inflammation, Dietary Omega 3, and Microbiota. Neural Plast. 2016;2016:3597209. doi: 10.1155/2016/3597209. Epub 2016 Oct 20. PMID: 27840741; PMCID: PMC5093279.

Cao X, Liu K, Liu J, Liu YW, Xu L, Wang H, Zhu Y, Wang P, Li Z, Wen J, Shen C, Li M, Nie Z, Kong XJ. Dysbiotic Gut Microbiota and Dysregulation of Cytokine Profile in Children and Teens With Autism Spectrum Disorder. Front Neurosci. 2021 Feb 10;15:635925. doi: 10.3389/fnins.2021.635925. PMID: 33642989; PMCID: PMC7902875.

Inulin:

Kellow NJ et al. Effect of dietary prebiotic supplementation on advanced glycation, insulin resistance and inflammatory biomarkers in adults with pre-diabetes: a study protocol for a double-blind placebo-controlled randomized crossover clinical trial. *BMC Endocrine Disorders*. 2014;14:55. https://www.ncbi.nlm.nih.gov/pubmed/25011647

Hopkins MJ, Macfarlane GT. Nondigestible Oligosaccharides Enhance Bacterial Colonization Resistance against *Clostridium difficile* In Vitro. *Applied and Environmental Microbiology*. 2003;69(4):1920-1927. https://www.ncbi.nlm.nih.gov/pmc/articles/PMC154806/

Collins S, Reid G. Distant Site Effects of Ingested Prebiotics. *Nutrients*. 2016;8(9):523. https://www.ncbi.nlm.nih.gov/pmc/articles/PMC5037510/

Slavin J. Significance of Inulin Fructans in the Human Diet. *Compre Rev in Food Science and Food Safety*. 2015 14;1: 37–47. http://onlinelibrary.wiley.com/doi/10.1111/1541-4337.12119/abstract

Microglia and Neuroinflammation:

Coomey R, Stowell R, Majewska A, Tropea D. The Role of Microglia in Neurodevelopmental Disorders and their Therapeutics. Curr Top Med Chem. 2020;20(4):272-276. doi: 10.2174/1568026620666200221172619. PMID: 32091337; PMCID: PMC7323119.

Petrelli F, Pucci L, Bezzi P. Astrocytes and Microglia and Their Potential Link with Autism Spectrum Disorders. *Frontiers in Cellular Neuroscience.* 2016;10:21. https://www.ncbi.nlm.nih.gov/pmc/articles/PMC4751265/

Norden, DM et al. Microglial Priming and Enhanced Reactivity to Secondary Insult in Aging, and Traumatic CNS Injury, and Neurodegenerative Disease. *Neuropharmacology* 96.0 0 (2015): 29–41. https://www.ncbi.nlm.nih.gov/pmc/articles/PMC4430467/

Calabrese, F et al. Brain-Derived Neurotrophic Factor: A Bridge between Inflammation and Neuroplasticity. *Frontiers in Cellular Neuroscience* 8 (2014): 430. https://www.ncbi.nlm.nih.gov/pmc/articles/PMC4273623/

Cunningham, Colm. Systemic Inflammation and Delirium – Important Co-Factors in the Progression of Dementia. *Biochemical Society Transactions* 39.4 (2011): 945–953. https://www.ncbi.nlm.nih.gov/pubmed/21787328

Paolicelli RC et al. Synaptic pruning by microglia is necessary for normal brain development. *Science* 2011 Sep 9;333(6048):1456-8. https://www.ncbi.nlm.nih.gov/pubmed/21778362

Omega Fatty Acids:

Mariamenatu AH, Abdu EM. Overconsumption of Omega-6 Polyunsaturated Fatty Acids (PUFAs) versus Deficiency of Omega-3 PUFAs in Modern-Day Diets: The Disturbing Factor for Their "Balanced Antagonistic Metabolic Functions" in the Human Body. J Lipids. 2021

Mar 17;2021:8848161. doi: 10.1155/2021/8848161. PMID: 33815845; PMCID: PMC7990530.

Simopoulos AP. The importance of the omega-6/omega-3 fatty acid ratio in cardiovascular disease and other chronic diseases. Exp Biol Med (Maywood). 2008 Jun;233(6):674-88. doi: 10.3181/0711-MR-311. Epub 2008 Apr 11. PMID: 18408140.

Madsen L, Kristiansen K. Of mice and men: Factors abrogating the anti-obesity effect of omega-3 fatty acids. *Adipocyte.* 2012;1(3):173-176. https://www.ncbi.nlm.nih.gov/pmc/articles/PMC3609096/

Reimers A, Ljung H. The emerging role of omega-3 fatty acids as a therapeutic option in neuropsychiatric disorders. *Ther Adv Psychopharmacol.* 2019;9:2045125319858901. Published 2019 Jun 24. doi:10.1177/2045125319858901

El-Ansary AK et al. On the protective effect of omega-3 against propionic acid-induced neurotoxicity in rat pups. *Lipids in Health and Disease.* 2011;10:142. https://www.ncbi.nlm.nih.gov/pmc/articles/PMC3170231/

Chang, P et al. Docosahexaenoic Acid (DHA): A Modulator of Microglia Activity and Dendritic Spine Morphology. *Journal of Neuroinflammation* 12 (2015): 34. https://www.ncbi.nlm.nih.gov/pmc/articles/PMC4344754/

Patterson E et al. Health Implications of High Dietary Omega-6 Polyunsaturated Fatty Acids. *Journal of Nutrition and Metabolism.* 2012;2012:539426. https://www.ncbi.nlm.nih.gov/pubmed/22570770

Harvey, LD. et al. Administration of DHA Reduces Endoplasmic Reticulum Stress-Associated Inflammation and Alters Microglial or Macrophage Activation in Traumatic Brain Injury. *ASN Neuro* 7.6 (2015): 1759091415618969. https://www.ncbi.nlm.nih.gov/pmc/articles/PMC4710127/

Liu, JJ. et al. Pathways of Polyunsaturated Fatty Acid Utilization: Implications for Brain Function in Neuropsychiatric Health and

Disease. *Brain research* 0 (2015): 220–246. https://www.ncbi.nlm.nih.gov/pmc/articles/PMC4339314/

Titos E et al. Resolvin D1 and its precursor docosahexaenoic acid promote resolution of adipose tissue inflammation by eliciting macrophage polarization toward an M2-like phenotype. *J Immun.* 2011 Nov 15;187(10):5408-18. https://www.ncbi.nlm.nih.gov/pubmed/22013115

Chen S et al. n-3 PUFA supplementation benefits microglial responses to myelin pathology. *Scientific Reports.* 2014;4:7458. https://www.ncbi.nlm.nih.gov/pubmed/25500548

Minkyung K et al. Impact of 8-week linoleic acid intake in soy oil on Lp-PLA2 activity in healthy adults. *Nutr & Metab.* 2017. 14:32. https://www.ncbi.nlm.nih.gov/pmc/articles/PMC5422895/

Christian LM et al. Body weight affects ω-3 polyunsaturated fatty acid (PUFA) accumulation in youth following supplementation in post-hoc analyses of a randomized controlled trial. *PLoS ONE.* 2017;12(4):e0173087. https://www.ncbi.nlm.nih.gov/pmc/articles/PMC5381773/

Igarashi M et al. Dietary N-6 Polyunsaturated Fatty Acid Deprivations Increases Docosahexaenoic Acid (DHA) in Rat Brain. *Journal of Neurochemistry.* 2012;120(6):985-997. https://www.ncbi.nlm.nih.gov/pmc/articles/PMC3296886/

Grundy T et al. Long-term omega-3 supplementation modulates behavior, hippocampal fatty acid concentration, neuronal progenitor proliferation and central TNF-α expression in 7 month old unchallenged mice. *Frontiers in Cellular Neuroscience.* 2014;8:399. https://www.ncbi.nlm.nih.gov/pmc/articles/PMC4240169/

Mazahery H, Stonehouse W, Delshad M, Kruger MC, Conlon CA, Beck KL, von Hurst PR. Relationship between Long Chain n-3 Polyunsaturated Fatty Acids and Autism Spectrum Disorder: Systematic Review and Meta-Analysis of Case-Control and Randomised Controlled Trials. Nutrients. 2017 Feb 19;9(2):155. doi: 10.3390/nu9020155. PMID: 28218722; PMCID: PMC5331586.

Prevention:

Chu DM et al. Maturation of the Infant Microbiome Community Structure and Function Across Multiple Body Sites and in Relation to Mode of Delivery. *Nature medicine.* 2017;23(3):314-326. https://www.ncbi.nlm.nih.gov/pubmed/28112736

Arslanoglu S et al. Early supplementation of prebiotic oligosaccharides protects formula-fed infants against infections during the first 6 months of life. *J Nutr.* 2007 Nov;137(11):2420-4. https://www.ncbi.nlm.nih.gov/pubmed/17951479

Helland IB et al. Maternal supplementation with very-long-chain n-3 fatty acids during pregnancy and lactation augments children's IQ at 4 years of age. *Pediatrics.* 2003 Jan;111(1):e39-44. https://www.ncbi.nlm.nih.gov/pubmed/12509593

Desai et al. Depletion of Brain Docosahexaenoic Acid Impairs Recovery from Traumatic Brain Injury. Annunziato L, ed. *PLoS ONE.* 2014;9(1):e86472. https://www.ncbi.nlm.nih.gov/pubmed/24475126

Carlson SE et al. DHA supplementation and pregnancy outcomes. *The American Journal of Clinical Nutrition.* 2013;97(4):808-815. https://www.ncbi.nlm.nih.gov/pubmed/23426033

Carvajal JA. Docosahexaenoic Acid Supplementation Early in Pregnancy May Prevent Deep Placentation Disorders. *BioMed Research International.* 2014;2014:526895. https://www.ncbi.nlm.nih.gov/pubmed/25019084

Fukuda H et al. Inhibition of sympathetic pathways restores postoperative ileus in the upper and lower gastrointestinal tract. *J Gastroenterol Hepatol.* 2007 Aug;22(8):12939. https://www.ncbi.nlm.nih.gov/pubmed/17688668

Perring S et al. Assessment of changes in cardiac autonomic tone resulting from inflammatory response to the influenza vaccination. *Clin Physiol Funct Imaging.* 2012 Nov;32(6):437-44. https://www.ncbi.nlm.nih.gov/pubmed/23031064

Jae SY et al. Does an acute inflammatory response temporarily attenuate parasympathetic reactivation? *Clin Auton Res.* 2010 Aug;20(4):229-33. https://www.ncbi.nlm.nih.gov/pubmed/20437076

De Wildt DJ et al. Impaired autonomic responsiveness of the cardiovascular system of the rat induced by a heat-labile component of Bordetella pertussis vaccine. *Infection and Immunity.* 1983;41(2):476-481. https://www.ncbi.nlm.nih.gov/pmc/articles/PMC264665/

Kashiwagi Y et al. Production of inflammatory cytokines in response to diphtheria-pertussis-tetanus (DPT), *haemophilus influenzae* type b (Hib), and 7-valent pneumococcal (PCV7) vaccines. *Human Vaccines & Immunotherapeutics.* 2014;10(3):677-685. https://www.ncbi.nlm.nih.gov/pmc/articles/PMC4130255/

Akiho H et al. Cytokine-induced alterations of gastrointestinal motility in gastrointestinal disorders. *World Journal of Gastrointestinal Pathophysiology.* 2011;2(5):72-81. https://www.ncbi.nlm.nih.gov/pmc/articles/PMC3196622/

Vantrappen G et al. The Interdigestive Motor Complex of Normal Subjects and Patients with Bacterial Overgrowth of the Small Intestine. *Journal of Clinical Investigation.* 1977;59(6):1158-1166. https://www.ncbi.nlm.nih.gov/pmc/articles/PMC372329/

Jacobs C et al. Dysmotility and PPI use are independent risk factors for small intestinal bacterial and/or fungal overgrowth. *Alimentary pharmacology & therapeutics.* 2013;37(11):1103-1111. https://www.ncbi.nlm.nih.gov/pmc/articles/PMC3764612/

Miyano Y et al. The Role of the Vagus Nerve in the Migrating Motor Complex and Ghrelin- and Motilin-Induced Gastric Contraction in Suncus. Covasa M, ed. *PLoS ONE.* 2013;8(5):e64777. https://www.ncbi.nlm.nih.gov/pmc/articles/PMC3665597/

Propionic Acid and Autism:

Choi J, Lee S, Won J, Jin Y, Hong Y, Hur TY, Kim JH, Lee SR, Hong Y. Pathophysiological and neurobehavioral characteristics of a propionic acid-mediated autism-like rat model. PLoS One. 2018 Feb 15;13(2):e0192925. doi: 10.1371/journal.pone.0192925. PMID: 29447237; PMCID: PMC5814017.

El-Ansary AK et al. Etiology of autistic features: the persisting neuro-toxic effects of propionic acid. *Journal of Neuroinflammation.* 2012;9:74. https://www.ncbi.nlm.nih.gov/pubmed/22531301

McFabe DF et al. Neurobiological effects of intraventricular propionic acid in rats possible role of short chain fatty acids on the pathogenesis and characteristics of autism spectrum disorders. *Behav Brain Res.* 2007. Jan 10:176(1);149-69. https://www.ncbi.nlm.nih.gov/pubmed/16950524

Xiong X, Liu D, Wang Y, Zeng T, Peng Y. Urinary 3-(3-Hydroxyphenyl)-3-hydroxypropionic Acid, 3-Hydroxyphenylacetic Acid, and 3-Hydroxyhippuric Acid Are Elevated in Children with Autism Spectrum Disorders. *BioMed Research International.* 2016. https://www.ncbi.nlm.nih.gov/pmc/articles/PMC4829699/

MacFabe DF. Short-chain fatty acid fermentation products of the gut microbiome: implications in autism spectrum disorders. *Microbial Ecology in Health and Disease.* 2012;23:10. https://www.ncbi.nlm.nih.gov/pubmed/23990817

Ferraris C, Meroni E, Casiraghi MC, Tagliabue A, De Giorgis V, Erba D. One Month of Classic Therapeutic Ketogenic Diet Decreases Short Chain Fatty Acids Production in Epileptic Patients. Front Nutr. 2021 Mar 29;8:613100. doi: 10.3389/fnut.2021.613100. PMID: 33855040; PMCID: PMC8039123.

Rifaximin:

Ponziani FR et al. Eubiotic properties of rifaximin: Disruption of the traditional concepts in gut microbiota modulation. *World Journal of Gastroenterology.* 2017;23(25):4491-4499. https://www.ncbi.nlm.nih.gov/pmc/articles/PMC3747729/

Gao, J et al. Rifaximin, gut microbes and mucosal inflammation: unraveling a complex relationship. Gut Microbes. 2014 Jul 1;5(4):571-5. https://www.ncbi.nlm.nih.gov/pubmed/25244596

Yao CK. The clinical value of breath hydrogen testing. *J Gastroenterologists Hepatol.* 2017 Mar;32 Suppl 1:20-22. https://www.ncbi.nlm.nih.gov/pubmed/28244675

Muniyappa P, Gulati R, Mohr F, Hupertz V. Use and safety of rifaximin in children with inflammatory bowel disease. J Pediatr Gastroenterol Nutr. 2009 Oct;49(4):400-4. doi: 10.1097/MPG.0b013e3181a0d269. PMID: 19668011.

Ghoshal UC et al. Utility of hydrogen breath tests in diagnosis of small intestinal bacterial overgrowth in malabsorption syndrome and its relationship with orocecal transit time. *Indian J Gastroenterol.* 2006 Jan-Feb;25(1):6-10. https://www.ncbi.nlm.nih.gov/pmc/articles/PMC4175689/

Muniyappa P et al. Use and safety of rifaximin in children with inflammatory bowel disease. *J Pediatricians Gastroenterol Nutr.* 2009 Oct;49(4):400-4. https://www.ncbi.nlm.nih.gov/pubmed/19668011

Pimentel M, Cash BD, Lembo A, Wolf RA, Israel RJ, Schoenfeld P. Repeat Rifaximin for Irritable Bowel Syndrome: No Clinically Significant Changes in Stool Microbial Antibiotic Sensitivity. *Digestive Diseases and Sciences.* 2017;62(9):2455-2463. https://www.ncbi.nlm.nih.gov/pmc/articles/PMC5561162/

Guslandi M. Rifaximin in the treatment of inflammatory bowel disease. World J Gastroenterol. 2011 Nov 14;17(42):4643-6. doi: 10.3748/wjg.v17.i42.4643. PMID: 22180705; PMCID: PMC3237300.

Vagus Nerve Stimulation:

van Hoorn A, Carpenter T, Oak K, Laugharne R, Ring H, Shankar R. Neuromodulation of autism spectrum disorders using vagal nerve stimulation. J Clin Neurosci. 2019 May;63:8-12. doi: 10.1016/j.jocn.2019.01.042. Epub 2019 Feb 4. PMID: 30732986.

Levy ML, Levy KM, Hoff D, Amar AP, Park MS, Conklin JM, Baird L, Apuzzo ML. Vagus nerve stimulation therapy in patients with autism spectrum disorder and intractable epilepsy: results from the vagus nerve stimulation therapy patient outcome registry. J Neurosurg Pediatr. 2010 Jun;5(6):595-602. doi: 10.3171/2010.3.PEDS09153. PMID: 20515333.

Yap JYY, Keatch C, Lambert E, Woods W, Stoddart PR, Kameneva T. Critical Review of Transcutaneous Vagus Nerve Stimulation: Challenges for Translation to Clinical Practice. Front Neurosci. 2020 Apr 28;14:284. doi: 10.3389/fnins.2020.00284. PMID: 32410932; PMCID: PMC7199464.

Badran BW, Jenkins DD, Cook D, Thompson S, Dancy M, DeVries WH, Mappin G, Summers P, Bikson M, George MS. Transcutaneous Auricular Vagus Nerve Stimulation-Paired Rehabilitation for Oromotor Feeding Problems in Newborns: An Open-Label Pilot Study. Front Hum Neurosci. 2020 Mar 18;14:77. doi: 10.3389/fnhum.2020.00077. PMID: 32256328; PMCID: PMC7093597.

Manning KE, Beresford-Webb JA, Aman LCS, Ring HA, Watson PC, Porges SW, Oliver C, Jennings SR, Holland AJ. Transcutaneous vagus nerve stimulation (t-VNS): A novel effective treatment for temper outbursts in adults with Prader-Willi Syndrome indicated by results from a non-blind study. PLoS One. 2019 Dec 3;14(12):e0223750. doi: 10.1371/journal.pone.0223750. PMID: 31794560; PMCID: PMC6890246.

Komegae EN, Farmer DGS, Brooks VL, McKinley MJ, McAllen RM, Martelli D. Vagal afferent activation suppresses systemic inflammation via the splanchnic anti-inflammatory pathway. Brain Behav Immun. 2018 Oct;73:441-449. doi: 10.1016/j.bbi.2018.06.005. Epub 2018 Jun 5. PMID: 29883598; PMCID: PMC6319822.

Koopman FA, Chavan SS, Miljko S, Grazio S, Sokolovic S, Schuurman PR, Mehta AD, Levine YA, Faltys M, Zitnik R, Tracey KJ, Tak PP. Vagus nerve stimulation inhibits cytokine production and attenuates disease severity in rheumatoid arthritis. Proc Natl Acad Sci U S

A. 2016 Jul 19;113(29):8284-9. doi: 10.1073/pnas.1605635113. Epub 2016 Jul 5. PMID: 27382171; PMCID: PMC4961187.

Marshall R, Taylor I, Lahr C, Abell TL, Espinoza I, Gupta NK, Gomez CR. Bioelectrical Stimulation for the Reduction of Inflammation in Inflammatory Bowel Disease. Clin Med Insights Gastroenterol. 2015 Dec 6;8:55-9. doi: 10.4137/CGast.S31779. PMID: 26692766; PMCID: PMC4671545.

Huston JM, Gallowitsch-Puerta M, Ochani M, Ochani K, Yuan R, Rosas-Ballina M, Ashok M, Goldstein RS, Chavan S, Pavlov VA, Metz CN, Yang H, Czura CJ, Wang H, Tracey KJ. Transcutaneous vagus nerve stimulation reduces serum high mobility group box 1 levels and improves survival in murine sepsis. Crit Care Med. 2007 Dec;35(12):2762-8. doi: 10.1097/01.CCM.0000288102.15975.BA. PMID: 17901837.

Zhang Q, Lu Y, Bian H, Guo L, Zhu H. Activation of the $\alpha7$ nicotinic receptor promotes lipopolysaccharide-induced conversion of M1 microglia to M2. Am J Transl Res. 2017 Mar 15;9(3):971-985. PMID: 28386326; PMCID: PMC5375991.

NOTES

ABOUT THE AUTHORS

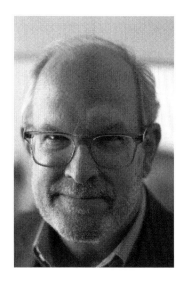

Dr. Patrick M. Nemechek, D.O. was born in Tucson, Arizona. He graduated with a B.S. in Microbiology from San Diego State University (1982) and obtained his Doctorate in Osteopathic Medicine from the University of Health Sciences, Kansas City, Missouri (1987).

Dr. Nemechek completed his training in internal medicine at UCLA School of Medicine (1990) where he had the distinguished honor of being named Chief Resident and later Clinical Instructor for the Department of Medicine at UCLA.

Dr. Nemechek's mentor at UCLA was Albert Einstein's nephew who encouraged him to go into the particularly complex field of HIV Medicine, which was the medical mystery of that time, where Dr. Nemechek would have the challenging freedom to save people's lives.

While at UCLA, Dr. Nemechek was recognized with the Robert S. Mosser Award for Excellence in Internal Medicine for his outstanding academic performance and instrumental role in starting UCLA's first HIV clinic at Kern Medical Center, Bakersfield, California.

In 1994, Dr. Nemechek moved to Kansas City, Missouri where he opened an HIV treatment and research facility named Nemechek Health Renewal.

It was at this point that Dr. Nemechek started work in earnest as a classically trained internal medicine "scientist-physician", entering the field of HIV when there was no diagnostic test, no treatment, and no answers.

Those early decades transformed Dr. Nemechek into an innovator who followed the latest research, looked at problems on a cellular and metabolic level, and became one of the first doctors develop treatment for wasting syndrome as well as other HIV-related complex problems.

Dr. Nemechek's innovative approach to the complexities of HIV disease garnered him honors such as being chosen as a "Site of Clinical Excellence" by Bristol Myers Squibb Company & KPMG Peat Marwick, being named one of the top HIV physicians in the U.S. by POZ magazine and receiving several nominations for the Small Business of the Year Award by the Greater Kansas City Chamber of Commerce.

During his 20 years in the Midwest, Dr. Nemechek authored, co-authored or co-collaborated on 72 scientific abstracts and publications, participated in 41 different clinical studies, and in 1999 became a founding investigator for the HIV Research Network, a consortium of 18 different universities and HIV treatment facilities funded by the U.S. Department of Health and Human Services.

He has served on numerous editorial, professional, and advisory boards as well as founding two non-profit HIV health advocacy organizations, the Bakersfield Aids Foundation and Fight Back KC.

By 2004, many of Dr. Nemechek's HIV patients were stable and leading normal lives but strangely they were starting to die of sudden cardiac events due to Cardiac Autonomic Neuropathy (CAN).

Dr. Nemechek set out to learn more about the lethal phenomena and in 2006 purchased new technology called spectral analysis that allowed him to tune into the communication signal between the heart and the brain, quantifying the balance and tone of the two branches of the autonomic nervous system.

Dr. Nemechek received additional training in autonomic testing and analysis at the Universidade De Lisboa, in Lisbon, Portugal, one of the top autonomic research facilities in the world.

Dr. Nemechek has now performed and analyzed thousands of autonomic patterns of damage. The more Dr. Nemechek learned about the field of Autonomic Medicine, the more he realized that it is the failure of the brain that sets into motion the failure of the body.

With his extensive research experience and expertise in metabolism, immunology, and the autonomic nervous system, Dr. Nemechek returned to his home state of Arizona in 2010 with his wife Jean and opened Nemechek Consultative Medicine, an Internal Medicine and Autonomic Medicine practice.

Jean Nemechek is uniquely qualified to run the business and co-author with Dr. Nemechek as she graduated with a B.A. in Communications and a B.S. in Journalism from the University of Kansas (1988, 1989) and a Juris Doctorate from Washburn School of Law (1993).

After relocating back home to Arizona, Dr. Nemechek was once again treating children and adults of all ages for routine matters. He was shocked at how incredibly sick the general population had become in just a few decades. The disease continuum had moved up about 40

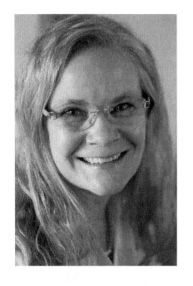

years it seemed, and diseases that had once struck only the elderly were routinely occurring in middle age or early adulthood.

Dr. Nemechek could recall when he was a medical student and his instructor called him into an exam room to see a person in their 50's who had diabetes. It was unheard of in those days to have someone "so young" with type II diabetes. Tragically, that disease is now quite commonplace in middle age as we have become collectively sick and old at an accelerated pace.

Dr. Nemechek realized that many of his routine patients were suffering from the early stages of disease and autonomic dysfunction (heartburn, headaches, fatigue), small intestine bacterial overgrowths – SIBO (intestinal distress, food intolerances), and their children were increasingly experiencing the symptoms arising from autonomic dysfunction and SIBO (anxiety, ADD, autism, and digestive and intestinal issues).

That is when Dr. Nemechek began, once again, to make history. He knew he had to change the practice of modern medicine back to the goals of healing the patient and reversing disease. Dr. Nemechek began to approach his regular patients with same the investigative research angle that he once did with HIV, he pushed beyond the disease labels to understand and resolve the underlying problem.

Dr. Nemechek started using all available scientific and medical tools to induce the nervous system and organs to repair themselves by normalizing inflammation control mechanisms, inducing natural stem cell production, and reactivating innate restorative mechanisms.

Starting in 2010, Dr. Nemechek embarked on an extraordinary path that involved altering and improving intestinal bacteria and reducing pro-inflammatory cytokines within the central nervous system and witnessed an unprecedented recovery in all five stages of autonomic dysfunction without long term medication. This is unheard of in our time.

As the years passed, Dr. Nemechek also began working with various current and former professional athletes whose brain symptoms resolved (Autonomic Advantage™ Brain Injury Recovery Program), and he began incorporating bioelectric medicine, specifically electro-modulation of the vagus nerve, with his patients.

Dr. Nemechek found the key to treatment and reversal of many of the common diseases affecting people today is reversing dysfunction of the autonomic nervous system in combination with the renewal of stem cell production and neurogenesis through the reduction of metabolic inflammation.

Because of his efforts and career experiences, Dr. Nemechek invented an effective program to prevent, reduce, or reverse autonomic nervous system damage through a combination of natural neuro-chemical supplements, short term prescription medications, dietary restrictions, and neuromodulation of the Vagus nerve.

Dr. Nemechek's treatment approach is extremely effective in the recovery of autonomic function from a variety of neuroinflammatory conditions including traumatic brain injury, concussion, chronic traumatic encephalopathy (CTE), post-concussion syndrome (PCS), Alzheimer's disease, Parkinson's disease, essential tremor, post-trau-matic stress disorder (PTSD), chronic depression, treatment-resistant epilepsy, autism, developmental delay, Asperger's syndrome, and sensory and motor disorders.

In 2016, Dr. Nemechek filed a patent application to protect his groundbreaking formula that is now known as "The Nemechek Protocol®" or The Nemechek Protocol for Autonomic Recovery (Patent No. 10,335,356).

In response to his unique expertise in clinical autonomics and the development of The Nemechek Protocol® for Autonomic Recovery, the practice was renamed (dba) Nemechek Autonomic Medicine in 2017.

This book explains the main tools used by Dr. Nemechek in his work with autistic and developmental delay patients in his medical practice using certain parts of The Nemechek Protocol®. His approach with these patients is now also commonly referred to as "The Nemechek Protocol for Autism", and it has spread throughout the world.

Made in the USA
Columbia, SC
16 June 2022

61797262R00172